THE Alexander TECHNIQUE WORKBOOK

THE Alexander
TECHNIQUE
WORKBOOK

*The Complete Guide
to Health, Poise and Fitness*

RICHARD BRENNAN

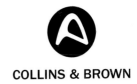

COLLINS & BROWN

First published in the United Kingdom
in 2011 by
Collins & Brown
10 Southcombe Street
London W14 0RA

An imprint of Anova Books Company Ltd

Distributed in the United States and Canada by
Sterling Publishing Co,
387 Park Avenue South, New York,
NY 10016-8810, USA

ISBN 978-1-84340-594-8

A CIP catalogue for this book is available from
the British Library.

10 9 8 7 6 5 4 3 2 1

Reproduction by Rival Colour UK Ltd.
Printed and bound by NPE Print Communications,
Singapore

This book can be ordered direct from the
publisher at www.anovabooks.com

CONTENTS
INTRODUCTION 6

*This book is dedicated to all those who
have the courage to take the risks necessary
to discover their True Self.*

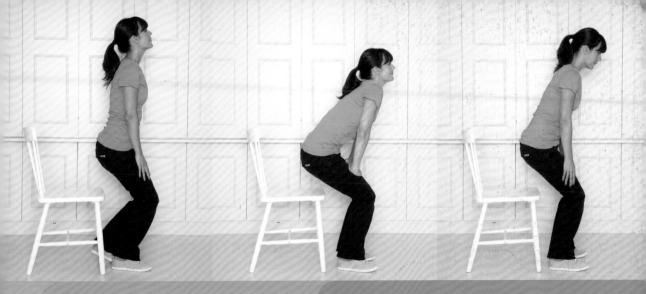

Introduction

To be what we are and to become what we are capable of becoming is the only end of life.

ROBERT LOUIS STEVENSON

It has been over 20 years since I wrote the first *Alexander Technique Workbook*, which has sold over 100,000 copies, and I have had many phone calls, e-mails and letters of appreciation thanking me for the book. For many, it was their first introduction to the Alexander Technique; some of those people are now Alexander teachers themselves.

The reason I wrote the book was to inform people about a very wonderful technique that had helped me a great deal when I was in a lot of pain with acute sciatica. My only regret was that I hadn't discovered it earlier. It changed my life so dramatically that after just a few lessons I applied to do the three-year Alexander teacher training programme. When I qualified as a teacher in 1989 I wanted to find a way of letting more people know about the Technique. At that time there were not very many easy to read books on the Alexander Technique, and this prompted me to write a book that could be understood by someone who knew nothing about the subject at all.

The Alexander Technique is a method of releasing the physical and mental tensions that many of us have accumulated throughout our lives. Often we are completely unaware of these tensions until we become ill and are unable to go on. They can contribute to headaches, backache, heart problems, arthritis and depression, as well as to a whole range of other ailments. If these unconscious muscular tensions are allowed to continue, as they often are, they can affect our quality of life by accelerating the ageing process and decreasing our vitality.

The ease and grace with which we move slowly become lost as we are burdened by more responsibilities. The Alexander Technique can help us to regain that poise and ease during even the most simple tasks. Our body is our most precious possession, yet we tend to give it the least attention – apart from when we are trying to look attractive. Without knowing it, we grossly interfere with our natural flow of movement to such an extent that many of

Val's story

Val Oatley
Age: 62 | Occupation: former ballet dancer

Val had arthritis in both her hands and feet, her shoulders and neck were in pain and she also suffered from chronic sciatica. After completing a course of day classes she had this to say:

'By means of the Alexander Technique I have acquired an awareness of where my body is in space, which means I am now able to control my muscle tension by means of my brain. This was essential if I was ever to maintain a posture without straining my body unconsciously.

I have discovered a completeness of my mind and body so that it can work as a whole entity, instead of as a jumble of separate limbs, head and torso all working independently of one another. This, of course, relieves a lot of unnecessary muscle tension and teaches me a way of restoring the completeness of the body in a relaxed and co-ordinated way that had been lost in my early childhood.

Most of my aches and pains have dropped away leaving me able to achieve a balance and poise not only of the body, but of the mind as well.'

us will at some time in our lives suffer from backache, solely due to poor posture. Yet there is nothing more attractive than someone who is moving in a balanced and co-ordinated way.

Few people are aware of the enormous benefits that the Alexander Technique offers and, as a result, many millions of people every year suffer needlessly. In this book I hope to explain the Alexander Technique as simply as possible and, through simple observation exercises and procedures, to show clearly how it can help you to enjoy a happier and more fulfilling life.

This new edition has been updated and added to without changing the easy style of the original book. The old line drawings have been replaced by colour photographs which I hope enhance the quality of the book. When the original book came out, hardly anyone had heard of the Internet and very few people owned a computer. In fact, I wrote the first book on a typewriter, which shows you how far we have progressed over two decades. I sincerely hope you enjoy this book, and find that it helps you to move through life with greater ease.

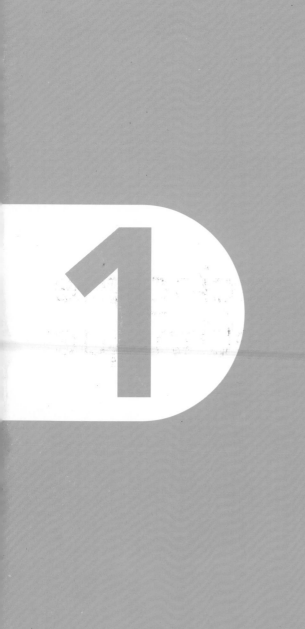

Introducing the Alexander Technique

1

What is the Alexander Technique?

Alexander established not only the beginnings of a far reaching science of the apparently involuntary movements we call reflexes, but a technique of correction and self-control which forms a substantial addition to our very slender resources in personal education.

GEORGE BERNARD SHAW, *LONDON MUSIC*

Since becoming an Alexander Technique teacher I have been interested in the different explanations of the Technique. Alexander's niece, Marjorie Barlow, said that the Alexander Technique is about 'knowing what you are doing, and making sure you can stop doing it if you so wish'. It can, however, take a lifetime to know exactly what you're doing, and that is what's so intriguing about the Technique. It can be described as a way of releasing muscle tension that may be the direct cause of a neck or back problem, but it is so much more. It is about learning about yourself and your reaction to what is going on around you. It is a technique based on awareness and choice.

A couple of years ago, I came across a passage in *A New Earth* by Eckhart Tolle which, to me, described what the Technique is really about. He was talking about the importance of all human beings needing to find a balance between the 'human' and the 'being' parts of themselves. Tolle went on to say that whatever we 'do' in this world belongs to a human dimension and, although it has a place and should be honoured, it will not be enough for a fulfilled and truly meaningful life. He clearly explains that the 'human' part is never enough, no matter how hard we try or what we achieve. Tolle then indicated that we often forget about the 'being' aspect of ourselves, which is found in the presence of consciousness, the consciousness that we all are, and that 'human' and 'being' are interwoven, not separate.

To me, this was an excellent description of what the Alexander Technique can offer. It helps you to put consciousness back into whatever you are doing; it is the practical application of being in the here and now. When you learn to be present by using the Technique you will be able to achieve the following:

- Move through life with greater ease.
- Become more aware of yourself: physically, mentally and emotionally.
- Prevent unnecessary wear and tear on your body.
- Detect excessive muscular tension in yourself and teach yourself how to let go of this unwanted tension.
- Stop wasting your energy and find new ways of moving more efficiently, thus avoiding fatigue at the end of the day.
- Recognize your behaviour patterns and change them if you wish.
- Become more conscious of your habitual ways of performing actions, thus allowing you to make more appropriate decisions.
- Rediscover the grace of movement you once had as a child.
- Be truly free.

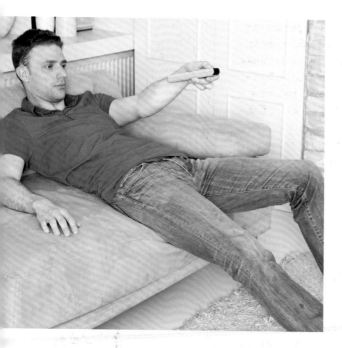

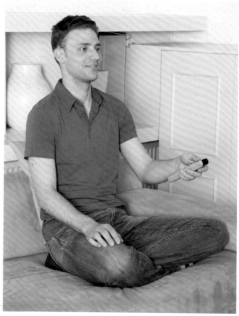

MOVING THROUGH LIFE WITH GREATER EASE

By applying the principles set out later in this book, you will be able to release habitual tensions and thus move in a very different way. This will make many of your everyday activities easier and allow you to enjoy life more fully. This in turn will affect the people around you. Your new-found happiness may rub off on to those you are close to. I often hear comments such as, 'Since my husband has had Alexander lessons he is a much nicer man to live with' or 'I feel much calmer and more relaxed since I have become involved in the Alexander Technique.'

Without realizing it, many of us make life more difficult than it really needs to be. We see it in others, but not so easily in ourselves. Life can soon become a joy, rather than the struggle so many of us make it.

⬆ The Alexander Technique offers awareness, balance and poise in everyday activities.

BECOMING MORE AWARE OF YOURSELF PHYSICALLY, EMOTIONALLY AND MENTALLY

This is the first step on the road to change. When you begin to become more aware of yourself you will be astounded at how much effort it used to take to perform very simple actions. A person can severely damage his or her back by picking up even a lightweight object, like a pen, from the floor. The main reason we do not notice the stress on our bodies is that our muscle tension increases by such minute amounts each day. Eventually, as this tension accumulates, it begins to interfere with the body's natural co-ordination and reflexes.

Since our body, mind and emotions are all inseparable, it follows that the way in which we move will in turn affect our mental and emotional wellbeing. Similarly, the way in which we feel or think will directly influence the way in which we undertake our daily activities.

PREVENTING UNNECESSARY WEAR AND TEAR ON YOUR BODY

By moving in a unco-ordinated manner or, as Alexander called it, 'misusing ourselves', the muscular and skeletal systems come under constant strain.

Some years ago, there was a newspaper account of an American woman on a visit to Britain who hired a car with a manual gearbox. She had only ever driven automatic cars and had no idea how to change gear. Consequently, she drove 190 km (120 miles) in first gear! She then complained to the rental company that the car didn't go very fast and was extremely noisy. Obviously, because she was not using the car correctly, both the engine and gearbox were under enormous strain and probably suffered permanent damage.

In the same way, if we do not use ourselves as nature intended (and so many people today do not), we may unknowingly be inflicting irreversible damage that will manifest later on in life. It is worth remembering that you can always exchange your car when it wears out, but you cannot exchange your body for a new one.

DETECTING AND RELEASING EXCESSIVE MUSCULAR TENSION

As you gradually become aware of yourself, you will begin to notice the muscular tensions I have mentioned. Certain muscles have become more and more tense while others become over-relaxed. This process takes place over many years and can eventually affect the physiological structure of the muscles. In fact, muscles can diminish in size and this is one of the reasons why older people seem to shrink.

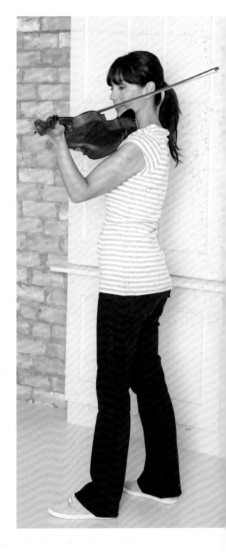

↑ The Technique can help musicians play their instruments without strain.

Most of us are completely ignorant of the effect this process has on our bodies until we experience pain. As our body ceases to function as it should, we visit the doctor hoping for answers she or he is often unable to give. We rarely ask ourselves, 'What am I doing to myself that could be causing this pain?'

If we could find the answer to this question, we would be able to stop doing it and the pain would ease naturally and soon disappear. However, because the tensions build up gradually over many years, the cause is often difficult to detect without help. Over many years we become so accustomed to certain stress levels in the body that we accept them as part of ourselves.

Letting go of these stresses is a relatively simple procedure once we have detected and recognized the reason for them.

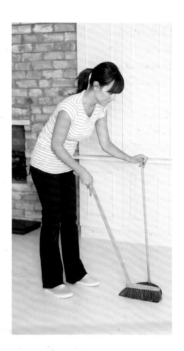

CONSERVING ENERGY BY FINDING NEW WAYS OF MOVING

The Alexander Technique will help you to stop and think before proceeding with your actions. This will allow you to do any activity with much greater efficiency of movement; in other words, to perform tasks with much less effort. This in turn can leave you with more energy to do the things you want to do. Many people experience more vitality which enhances their life. Young children seem to have endless reserves of energy. This is partly because they use their bodies in a graceful and co-ordinated way and do not waste energy as many adults do.

RECOGNIZING AND CHANGING YOUR PATTERNS OF BEHAVIOUR

As we have said, throughout life we all develop physical, mental and emotional patterns of behaviour. Other people are often more aware of these patterns in our behaviour than we are ourselves. We will respond to a given stimulus in a set way, irrespective of whether or not it is appropriate to the situation. As many of these patterns are below our level of consciousness, we will repeat them again and again without realizing what we are doing.

The Alexander Technique will enable you to bring these habitual behavioural tendencies into consciousness – which can give you a chance to change them, especially if they are having a detrimental effect on your wellbeing. The implications are far-

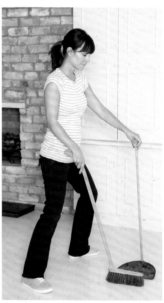

⬆ Learning to perform simple activities with better 'use' can reduce tension and ease pain.

reaching because you will be able to behave in an appropriate way in any situation that life presents, thus avoiding stress or illness later on.

RECOGNIZING AND CHANGING YOUR HABITUAL WAYS OF PERFORMING ACTIONS

Many of us, in Western civilization, use our bodies in a clumsy and awkward manner. We often perform our actions in a stereotyped way, and these habits feel 'right' to us, regardless of the strain they put on our structure. In this way, by placing excessive demands on ourselves, serious damage may be caused to our bodies. Many thousands of people suffer from a prolapsed intervertebral disc (more commonly known as a slipped disc). This is often caused by constant repetition of bending down in such a way that the spine is put under strain. The pressure is so great that the intervertebral disc is caught in a vice between the two adjacent vertebrae and literally 'squeezed' out of place (see Chapter 12).

By simply stopping for a moment to find the easiest way of performing any action, we not only avoid inflicting an unnecessary burden upon ourselves, but we may also save ourselves a great deal of time in the long run. Old proverbs such as 'Look before you leap' or 'More haste, less speed' are very appropriate in this fast-moving world in which we find ourselves.

RECREATING THE GRACE OF MOVEMENT YOU HAD AS A CHILD

The Alexander Technique is not so much a process of learning, but more a way of remembering what we have long since forgotten. It could be defined as a process of unlearning or re-education of the entire psycho-physical functioning of the human being.

Alexander himself often said that if you stop doing what is wrong, then the right thing will happen automatically. In other words, when we stop interfering with the natural reflexes and co-ordination of the body, then the body will perform with optimum efficiency and with greater ease of movement.

No matter what our age, we can regain some of that graceful, poised way of being that we see so clearly in young children, which is still latent in each and every one of us. I have taught pupils up to the age of 84 who have benefited from a course of lessons. Even

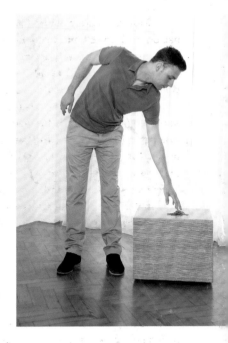

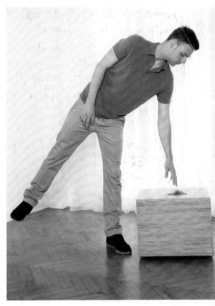

↑ Being in balance when picking up an object will reduce muscle tension.

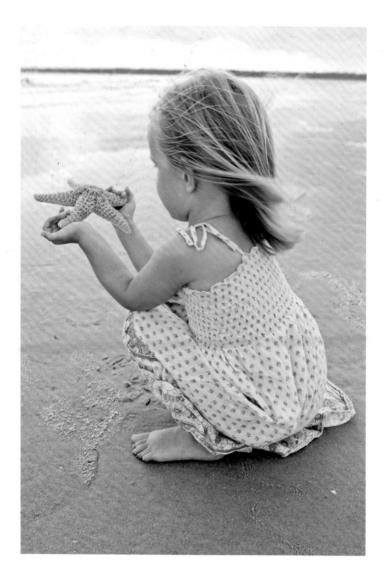

← Children have a natural balance and co-ordination in all actions they perform.

very elderly people are able to move more freely and can do far more without becoming fatigued.

When he was in his 80s, George Bernard Shaw had Alexander Technique lessons from Frederick Alexander himself. Shaw could not climb the three steps up to Alexander's front door without help when he went for his first lesson. After a course of lessons he was able to move around without help, and into his 90s he was thought

Caroline's story

Caroline Green
Age: 27 | Occupation: computer programmer/analyst

I had been suffering from intermittent lower back pain and neck ache for some years. I could not understand what it was that was causing the problem. I ate well, meditated regularly and practised Tai Chi, so I was convinced that I had retained a reasonable posture. I had also become aware that my breathing was often shallow and fast, and that there was a basic lack of ease throughout my body. However, awareness alone did not eradicate the problem, so nothing changed and I began to feel stuck. What I had failed to consider was that my lifestyle and my attitude to life could be part of the problem.

I grew up believing, like so many other people, that success and money were the two most important things in life, even at the cost of just being myself. I was heading for promotion after promotion in my job, but where was this happiness that I had been promised? I was becoming more miserable because I was trying to be someone else rather than just myself.

I heard about the Alexander Technique, started to have some lessons, and was amazed at the remarkable effect. I left my first lesson feeling light, free of tension and more full of energy than I had for a long time. My teacher said this was how my body could feel if it were not so bound up with the physical tension resulting from harmful postural habits. I realized that these habits had been caused by the unhealthy emotional and psychological attitudes that had been imposed on me by society. I noticed that I had a persistent habit of slumping when I sat and that my shoulders were curving in toward each other – this was caused by a basic lack of confidence that had been with me through my childhood. As I began to expand the upper part of my chest, I automatically began to have more confidence in myself and, after subsequent lessons, there were many other psychological changes that went hand in hand with the physical ones.

I have begun to understand how my body works, and when I feel pain I recognize it as a signal for me to stop and listen to what it is trying to tell me. I have learned how to perform even simple tasks in a different way so as not to put undue stress on myself. I still suffer from a little back pain from time to time, but I can now eradicate it in a matter of minutes by lying in the recommended position. It was a revelation to me that I did not have to be a victim of pain and I could do something for myself to get rid of it. I no longer accept tension and pain as inevitable and this makes me feel much more in control of my life.

of by friends and acquaintances as very sprightly. In fact, he died at the age of 94 after falling off a ladder while pruning a tree, and not many 94 year olds are able to climb ladders at all.

To start moving in these new ways, we need to become aware of the extent to which we interfere with many of our body's natural processes, including the respiratory, nervous and circulatory systems. Our children can, in fact, be our greatest teachers.

Spending a few moments watching a child aged three or four playing on the beach or in the park can show us much about the way our bodies were originally designed to be used. This is quite different from the way in which we become accustomed to using our bodies in our later years.

Most people report a feeling of lightness and a greater sense of wellbeing after just one or two Alexander lessons. At first this sensation is only temporary, but with further lessons it can become permanent.

BECOMING FREE

As a result of Alexander's observations, both about himself and others, he became increasingly convinced that the body, the mind, the emotions and the spirit not only influence each other, but are completely inseparable and that, if any one of these is misused, the other three will be affected.

It is not difficult to see that the way we think directly affects the way we feel and that this, in turn, affects our general performance in life. In any line of work, a person who is happy will often do a job much better than when they are unhappy. Our successes and our apparent failures lead us to think of ourselves in a certain way. Equally, when we learn to develop a new freedom in the way we move, we will also be able to free our thoughts from preconceived ideas and fixed prejudices and will be able to think and feel differently about many issues in our lives. This process will ultimately guide us to the freedom of our spirit, bringing us a sense of happiness and fulfilment which we may not have enjoyed since childhood.

Throughout history, men and women have given their lives for the freedom of family or country, yet few realize that they are trapped by the habitual way they think and are imprisoned by the growing pressures inflicted upon them daily. This is not to say we should live outside the rules we have set for ourselves, but rather that we should consciously choose not to react in a way that is detrimental to ourselves or to those around us.

The actual practice of the Alexander Technique is set down clearly and simply in the following chapters of this book, but it is useful at this stage to see what it does and does not offer.

In short, the Alexander Technique is something we learn in order to help ourselves, rather than a treatment whereby a doctor or therapist 'does something' to the patient.

Defining the Alexander Technique

THE TECHNIQUE IS

- A way of understanding how the body is naturally designed to work.
- A method of heightening our awareness, both of ourselves and the world around us.
- A re-education of how to use the body in such a way that our psycho-physical equilibrium can be restored.
- A process that can help us to recognize the interference that we ourselves inflict upon the body's natural functions.
- A way to use our thinking capacity to bring about a desired change so that we may go about our daily activities in a more co-ordinated fashion.
- A way of expanding our level of awareness.
- A technique that helps us to choose more consciously.
- A technique that we can practise on our own to help us move in a way that carries the minimum amount of tension at any given time. (Note: obviously we need a certain amount of tension to function; the trouble is we often over-do it.)

THE TECHNIQUE IS NOT

- A therapy.
- A form of treatment of any kind.
- Anything to do with massage, or the like.
- A form of healing – although the body's natural healing processes may well be activated.
- An exercise programme in any shape or form.
- Manipulation.
- A complementary medicine, such as homoeopathy, acupuncture or osteopathy. You do not have to be ill or have something wrong with you to benefit from the Technique. It is just that many of us start to look at the way we live only in times of crisis and it is worth reminding ourselves that prevention is better than cure.

2

How it Evolved

*The real voyage of discovery
consists not in seeking new
landscapes but in having new eyes.*

MARCEL PROUST

When beginning to learn the Alexander Technique, it can be very useful to understand how Alexander made the discoveries about himself, and the way he developed this method of teaching other people.

A LITTLE HISTORY

Frederick Matthias Alexander was born in Australia on 20 January 1869. He spent his childhood in Wynyard, a small town on the north-west coast of Tasmania. The eldest of eight children born to John and Betsy Alexander, Alexander was born prematurely and was not expected to live more than a few weeks. It was only his mother's overwhelming love for her child that ensured his survival. She was in fact the local nurse and midwife.

Throughout his childhood, Alexander was plagued by one illness or another, mainly nasal and other respiratory difficulties.

↓ **Frederick Matthias Alexander (1869–1955).**

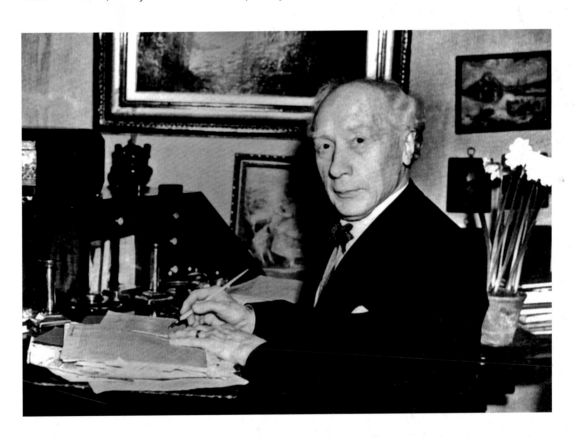

Although he started school, he was soon taken away because of his ill health and was given private tuition in the evenings by the local school teacher. This left Alexander with plenty of free time during the day to spend with his father's horses. Gradually he became expert at training and managing them, and in this way acquired the sensitivity of touch which was to prove invaluable later on.

At the age of nine or 10 Alexander's health began to improve and, at the age of 17, financial pressures within the family forced him to leave the outdoor life he had grown to love, to work in the office of a tin-mining company in the nearby town of Mount Bischoff. In his spare time he developed an interest in amateur dramatics and playing the violin.

By the time he was 20, Alexander had saved up enough money to travel to Melbourne where he stayed with his uncle, and for three months spent all his hard-earned money experiencing the best in theatre, art and music. By the end of his visit he had decided to train as a reciter.

To finance his training, which he did in the evenings and at weekends, Alexander took various jobs: working in an estate agent's office, in a large department store and as a tea taster for a firm of tea merchants. He quickly established an excellent reputation as an actor and reciter, and soon formed his own theatre company, specializing in one-man Shakespeare recitals. He was particularly fond of *The Merchant of Venice* and *Hamlet*.

VOICE PROBLEMS

Before long, the respiratory troubles that had plagued Alexander as a young child returned. His voice became hoarse and, on one occasion, he completely lost his voice during a performance. Soon he was reluctant to accept engagements for fear of losing his voice at a crucial moment in front of an audience. Seeking advice from doctors and voice trainers, he was given medication and was instructed to rest his voice and to gargle. But these solutions gave only temporary relief.

The career he loved was in jeopardy and he was willing to try anything to find a cure. Finally, one of his doctors prescribed a complete rest of the voice for a full two weeks before his next recital. The doctor assured him that if he followed these instructions to the letter his voice would return to normal.

By this time Alexander was so desperate that he hardly spoke at all during that time, and when he returned to the stage he was delighted to find that the hoarseness had completely disappeared. His delight soon turned to distress, however, because before he was even halfway through the performance the voice problem had returned and, by the end of the evening, the hoarseness was so acute that he could hardly speak. Alexander's disappointment was beyond words when he realized he could never look forward to more than temporary relief and would thus be forced to give up a career to which he was deeply committed and which promised to be highly successful.

The next day he went back to the same doctor, whose only advice was that he should persevere with the treatment. 'But', said Alexander, 'if my voice was perfect at the beginning of my recital, yet had deteriorated so much that by the end I could barely speak, is it not fair to conclude that it was something I was doing that evening in using my voice that was the cause of the trouble?'

The doctor thought for a moment, and then agreed, thus prompting Alexander to enquire: 'Can you tell, then, what it was I did that caused the trouble?' The doctor frankly admitted that he could not. 'Very well, if that is so,' Alexander replied, 'I must try and find out for myself.'

This dialogue between Alexander and his doctor is at the heart of the technique he was to go on to develop. It became his firm conviction that, if we suffer from headaches, backache, arthritis, insomnia or other ailments, there must always be a cause at the root of the problem. This is actually a modification of the well-known physical law of cause and effect, namely that every action has an opposite reaction. Alexander had experienced the reaction as the loss of his voice. Now he needed to discover the action that was causing this phenomenon.

THE QUEST BEGINS

It is important to remember that it was Alexander's overriding passion for the theatre that gave him the unswerving determination to see his task through in spite of the many setbacks along the way.

The story that follows is a tale of exploration, an important voyage of discovery of one man which led him to find the fundamental workings of the body. It is a complex journey and it may take at least two or three readings of this section to become acquainted with Alexander's way of thinking and the basic principles upon which his Technique is based.

All these principles are explained in detail throughout the rest of the book, so I suggest you might like to re-read this section again at the end.

After Alexander's conversation with his doctor, he was left with only two leads: one was his observation that the hoarseness in his voice appeared when he was reciting and the second was that, when he rested his voice, or was confined to ordinary talking, the hoarseness disappeared.

The journey had begun. He began to observe himself minutely in the mirror, first while he was speaking in an ordinary voice, and then while he was reciting some Shakespeare. He repeated the experiment many times and found that while he was merely speaking he noticed nothing unusual, but when he was reciting he saw that three things were happening:

- He tended to pull back his head onto the spine.
- He depressed his larynx (the area of the throat containing the vocal cords).
- He began to suck in breath through the mouth in a way that produced a gasping sound.

After noting these tendencies he watched himself again during ordinary speech and found he was doing exactly the same three actions, but to a much lesser degree, which was why he had not perceived them before. When he discovered this marked difference between what he did in ordinary speaking and what he did in reciting, he realized he had a definite clue which might explain things and thus he was encouraged to explore further.

The next step was to find a way to prevent or change these damaging tendencies, and here he found himself in a maze. He asked himself the following questions:

- Was it the sucking in of the breath that caused the pulling back of the head and the depressing of the larynx?
- Was it the pulling back of the head that caused the depressing of the larynx and the sucking in of breath?
- Was it the depressing of the larynx that caused the sucking in of the breath and the pulling back of the head?

> If you will do what I did, you will be able to do what I do.
> **FREDERICK MATTHIAS ALEXANDER**

He was unable to answer these questions at first, so he went on patiently experimenting in front of the mirror. After some time he realized that he was unable directly to prevent the sucking in of air or the depression of the larynx, but that he could to some extent prevent the pulling back of the head. This led to an even more important discovery – namely, that when he did succeed in preventing the pulling back of his head, this indirectly lessened the sucking in of air and eased the pressure on the larynx.

At this point he wrote in his journal:

> The importance of this discovery cannot be over-estimated, for through it I was led on to the further discovery of the primary control of the working of all the mechanisms of the human organism, and this marked the first important stage of my investigation.

It is important here to take a break from the story to clarify what Alexander meant by the 'primary control'.

THE PRIMARY CONTROL

The Primary Control acts as the main organizer of the body. It governs the working of all our mechanisms and so renders the control of our complex human organism comparatively simple. It is the dynamic relationship between our head and the rest of our body, and is often referred to as 'the head-neck-back relationship'. It is important to point out that this relationship is not one of position, but one of freedom of each to the other.

When, due to excess muscle tension, the head is pulled back and down, the Primary Control is interfered with. This, in turn, can interfere with other reflexes throughout the body, and can result in a lack of co-ordination and balance. A good example of this can be seen in horse riding. When a rider wishes to stop the horse in an emergency, he or she pulls the horse's head back with the reins and the animal immediately loses its co-ordination and soon comes to a standstill. It can also be demonstrated on a pet cat: if the cat's head is gently tipped in a backward direction the cat cannot function properly until it re-establishes control over its head, neck and back in relation to each other.

After his initial discovery of the Primary Control, Alexander noted further that when he was able to prevent the misuse of his head and larynx, the hoarseness in his voice decreased accordingly. When he was later examined by the medical profession, there was a considerable improvement in the condition of his vocal cords and larynx. This confirmed his suspicion that the way he 'used' himself had a marked effect on the functioning of his respiration and voice. (Alexander was extremely precise in the words and phrases he used to describe his new discoveries. For example, a term like 'using himself' may sound strange, but it is more correct than 'using his body', since he was talking about using his whole self and not just his body.)

The second major observation was: *the way in which he used himself directly affected the functioning of his body and therefore affected his performance.*

After giving the matter some thought, Alexander concluded that if he put his head even further forward he might influence the functioning of his voice still more as a way of eliminating the hoarseness altogether. So he proceeded to 'put' his head forward. He found, however, that past a certain point he tended once again to pull his head down as well as forward, which in turn had the same damaging effect on his vocal and respiratory organs.

Alexander continued to experiment over a long period of time, and this led him to see that, by using his head and neck in this way, there was also a tendency to lift his chest and shorten his whole stature. This observation had far-reaching implications, as we shall presently see.

The next important observation was: *pulling back his head affected his whole structure.*

Alexander experimented still further and noticed that his tendency to lift the chest also caused him to increase the arch of his spine which, in turn, narrowed his back. This led him to the conclusion that: *the misuse he had noticed was not just of specific parts (as first presumed) but of his whole being.*

He then examined the effect that shortening and lengthening had on his voice. He found that the best results (that is, when he was least hoarse) happened when he lengthened his stature. In *trying* to do this, however, he found that he shortened more often than he lengthened. Looking for an explanation for this, he saw that he had a tendency to pull his head down as well as back. Thus, he realized that in order to maintain a lengthened structure: *he must put his head forward and up.*

Alexander believed he had finally solved his problem, but this was not yet the case. When it came to reciting, while trying to put his head forward and up, he noticed that he was still lifting his chest, arching his spine and narrowing his back. This made him suspect that what he *thought* he was doing and what he was actually doing were two different things entirely.

At this stage in the proceedings he brought in two other mirrors, one on each side of the original. With their aid he could see that his suspicions were justified and that, when he attempted to maintain a lengthening in stature and speak at the same time, he actually pulled his head back (and not forward as he had intended). He had just stumbled upon what he later called Faulty Sensory Appreciation.

FAULTY SENSORY APPRECIATION

In simple terms, this means that the sensory feedback system that informs us where we are in space in relation to the earth may sometimes be untrustworthy. This also applies to the relationship of one part of our body to another. As in Alexander's case, what we *feel* we are doing may in fact be the opposite of what we are actually doing. This is probably the biggest pitfall when learning the Technique, and I will come back to this subject later (see pages 64–75).

Alexander was very disturbed at this point. Even though he had located the cause of his problem and believed he had found the remedy, he was unable to make use of it because he could not carry out the actions he had intended. He carefully reviewed the situation and decided there was nothing for it but to persevere.

He continued experimenting on himself month after month with both successes and failures. He began to notice a great deal of undue muscle tension, particularly in his legs, feet and toes. His toes were contracted and bent downwards in such a way as made his feet unduly arched and threw the weight of his body onto the outside of his feet. Naturally, this adversely affected his whole balance. Alexander became more and more convinced that the abnormal amount of muscle tension in his legs and feet was indirectly associated with the loss of his voice.

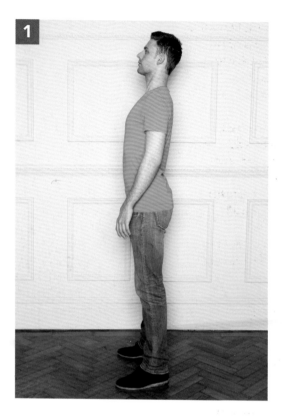

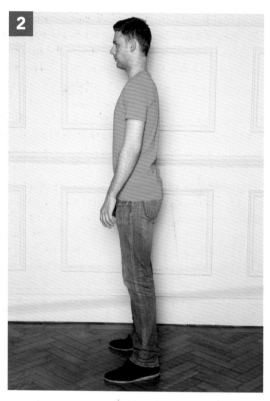

DIRECTIONS

It slowly dawned on Alexander that his efforts up until now had been misdirected and this led him to ask: 'What is this direction upon which I have been depending?' He had to admit that he had never thought about how he directed himself but had used himself in a way that felt natural to him.

He stopped at this point to examine all the information he had acquired so far. The particular issues he had noted were:

- That the pulling of his head back and down when he felt that he was putting it forward and up was proof that the movement of the particular parts concerned was being misdirected and that this misdirection was connected with his untrustworthy feelings.
- That this misdirection was unconscious and, together with the associated untrustworthy feeling, was part and parcel of his habitual use of himself.

↑ 1. Trying to stand up straight can often cause a person to actually lean backward.
2. People often find that when standing straight they feel like they are too far forward.

- That this unconscious misdirection leading to a wrong habitual use of himself, including in particular the incorrect use of his head and neck, came into play as the result of a decision to use his voice. In other words, this misdirection was an instinctive response to the stimulus to use his voice.

The next step was to discover which direction would be necessary to bring about a new and improved use of the head and neck, therefore indirectly influencing the larynx, the breathing and other mechanisms of the body.

Alexander saw that, if he was ever to react satisfactorily when using his voice, he must replace his old instinctive (unreasoned) habits with a new, conscious (reasoned) use of himself. While reciting he started consciously to 'direct' himself in such a way as to correct his old inappropriate habits. He was immediately confronted by a series of startling and unexpected experiences:

- He found no clear dividing line between reasoned and unreasoned directions.
- He was successful in using himself in a new improved way until the point of actually speaking, when he reverted to his old habitual use.
- As soon as he attempted to gain an end (that is, reciting), his unconscious habits dominated his reasoned directions, which he called 'orders'.

Alexander was extremely disappointed at these findings. Although he was making many discoveries from his experiments, he seemed to be unable to change the way in which he used himself while reciting. In exasperation, he gave up trying to 'do' anything to gain his end, and at last saw that, if he was ever to control his instinctive unconscious habits, he must at first refuse to 'do' anything immediately in response to the stimulus of speaking. He called this 'inhibition'.

INHIBITION

Alexander realized that, by giving up and not trying to do anything, and by merely thinking of his direction, he had achieved what he had been trying to do for several years. In other words, simply by thinking of his head going forward and upwards he prevented the pulling back of the head which, in turn, lengthened his stature and produced a beneficial effect on his larynx and vocal cords. Alexander eventually came up with a plan that involved using inhibition and direction which he practised over and over again until it produced the results he had been looking for.

At this point he wrote:

> After I had worked on this plan for a considerable time, I became free from my tendency to revert to my wrong habitual use in reciting, and the marked effect of this upon my functioning convinced me that I was at last on the right track, for once free from this tendency, I also became free from the throat and vocal trouble and from the respiratory and nasal difficulties with which I had been beset from birth.

So, as so often happens, Alexander had stumbled almost accidentally on some crucial information about the functioning of the body and about how we interfere with many of our processes without even realizing we are doing so. When Alexander first noticed that he interfered with his body reflexes by pulling his head back and down, he thought this was merely a personal idiosyncrasy. Later, through teaching others, he realized that in fact this interference was practically universal to the whole of modern civilization.

DEVELOPING THE TECHNIQUE

After finding the solution to his problem, word soon spread about Alexander's success in 'curing' himself, and many actors and reciters began to seek his advice. He began to realize that with the gentle guidance of his hands he could correct other people's many and varied ailments.

Although he resumed his career of acting and reciting, he also began to take on pupils and to teach them his Technique on a professional basis. At this point he was joined by his younger brother, Albert Redden Alexander, and together they worked out various procedures and instructions which were incorporated into the Technique. The two brothers worked together for about six years, teaching in Sydney and Melbourne.

The practice continued to grow as the emphasis began to shift away from voice development and on to the control of reactions throughout the whole body. Several doctors began referring their patients to the Alexander brothers. One of them, Dr J. W. Stewart McKay, a prominent surgeon in Sydney, persuaded Alexander to go to London in order to bring the Technique before a larger public.

He left Australia for good in the spring of 1904 and, with only a reference of introduction from Dr McKay, he soon set up a practice in Victoria Street, and later moved to 16 Ashley Place, in the centre of London.

Alexander soon established his teaching methods and became something of a cult figure. He taught many prominent figures, among them George Bernard Shaw, Aldous Huxley, the actor Sir Henry Irving, Sir Charles Sherrington, Nobel prize-winner for physiology and medicine, and Professor E. Coghill, anatomist and physiologist.

Alexander continued to practice in London until war broke out in 1914, when he set sail for the United States and established his Technique there. For a time, he spent alternate six-month periods in Britain and America. By 1925 he had settled back in London, and set up a school to teach his Technique to children. This school carried on until 1934, when it moved to Bexley in Kent.

THE ALEXANDER TECHNIQUE TRAINING COURSE

By the time Alexander had reached the age of 60, he was under pressure from many quarters to set up a training school for teachers in case he died before leaving an heir to carry on his work. In 1931 he set up the first Alexander Technique Training Course in his home at Ashley Place. He went on teaching privately as well as training teachers until his death in October 1955.

Since his death, the Technique has become famous throughout the world as more and more people turn to it in the hope of finding a solution to problems when often all else has failed.

3

The Benefits of the Alexander Technique

We already notice, with growing amazement, very striking improvements in such diverse things as high blood pressure, breathing, depth of sleep, overall cheerfulness and mental alertness, resilience against outside pressures, and in such a refined skill as playing a musical instrument.

PROFESSOR NIKOLAAS TINBERGEN, NOBEL PRIZE-WINNER FOR MEDICINE AND PHYSIOLOGY 1973, ACCEPTANCE SPEECH

The Alexander Technique is a very simple yet profound way of becoming more aware of the balance, posture and co-ordination of our bodies as we perform our numerous everyday activities. This subsequently allows us to be more aware of the excessive muscular tension that most of us unknowingly hold within our bodies. This undetected tension gradually builds up over many years, and later on in life may result in stiffness, pain and even deformities, which we often accept as an inevitable part of old age.

At first it is difficult to comprehend that the deterioration we take for granted is neither normal nor inevitable. And, because we are led to believe that so many of our aches and pains are caused by general wear and tear, many of us do little to find a remedy for them. We put up with the discomfort without question, and when our doctors say, 'This is what you must expect at your age', this merely confirms what we think already.

Some time ago, a woman in her mid-50s came to me for Alexander Technique lessons. She had been to see her doctor about a very painful right knee. After many tests the doctor explained to her that she had arthritis of the knee. She asked the doctor to explain what arthritis is and was told that it is normal wear and tear on the joints and, since she was over 50, she needed to accept it. She was confused and said to the doctor 'but I have two knees and, as far as I am aware, they are both exactly the same age. How is it that one is worn and torn and the other is perfectly okay?' During her Alexander lessons she was able to see that she had the habit of standing on her right leg and that this was the root of the problem. She learned to stand more evenly on both feet and, within a short time, the pain in her knee was gone.

Many of our ailments are directly caused or exacerbated by poor posture, which can be avoided if we use our bodies in a co-ordinated way throughout our life. Pain is nature's last resort – its way of informing us that something is wrong. Yet there are many other signals earlier on which we either tend to ignore or are unaware of. And, even when we are in a great deal of pain, instead of listening to what our body is trying to tell us, we tend to block out the symptoms with a variety of pain-killing drugs. If we asked ourselves what it is that causes so much physical suffering in our modern civilization, we might then gain an insight into how we could sit, stand or move in a less stressful way, in order to relieve our aches and pains.

These days, good posture is rare. The way in which we hold our bodies is the result of an accumulation of life's past experiences – physical, emotional and mental. We become trapped in certain postures, not realizing that the rigid shape we have acquired is unnatural or that it can lead to ill health in the future. An example of this is depression. One can see that people who collapse down into themselves could end up suffering from depression at some point, whereas, if they were to stand or sit in a more upright or poised manner, they would not tend to suffer from depression.

REASONS WHY OUR POSTURE CHANGES WITH AGE

- Many hours of sitting at school.
- Lack of exercise.
- Our fear reflex is constantly and inappropriately stimulated.
- The speed with which we often have to accomplish our tasks.
- The goal-oriented attitude that we are taught as children and at work.
- A distinct lack of interest in the present.
- The development of habits, both physical and mental.

MANY HOURS OF SITTING AT SCHOOL

In his early years, a child moves freely and naturally. If you observe the posture of a four-year-old child then that of a 16-year-old adolescent, you will find very obvious and startling differences. The four-year-old will be more upright in a natural and effortless way, whereas the 16-year-old will be much more slumped and, in order to keep himself erect while standing or sitting, will invariably tense his lower back. This will cause a shortening of the whole structure.

This process often begins within a few months of starting school. Any primary school teacher will tell you that young children do not want to sit still, yet it is the only way to maintain order in the classroom. Sitting for a short while is fine, especially when it is the child's free choice, but the number of hours that children have to sit increases with age until, in the early teens, a child can sit for as many as 10 hours a day when homework, time in front of a computer and television are taken into consideration. This is harmful on two accounts:

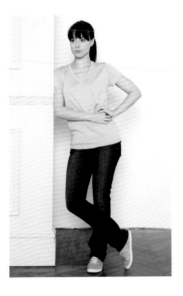

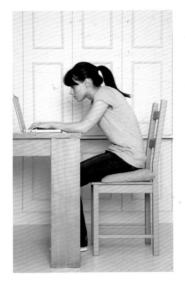

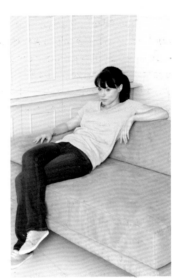

- Holding the body still for any length of time causes the tiring and consequently tensing of numerous muscles.
- The design of chairs in general does not take into account the mechanics of the human structure. The natural tendency for everyone is to collapse down into a slumped position while sitting in chairs or sofas.

↑ Many of the ways we sit and stand can put the muscular system under unnecessary stress.

It is also important to realize that the spine can be under greater pressure when sitting than in almost any other position.

If you observe children carefully, you will notice they sink down into themselves each time their minds start to wander. Because of the exorbitant number of hours we spend sitting, this slumped position becomes the norm and thus crystallizes into our habitual way of being.

An average child who starts school at the age of five and leaves at the age of 18 will probably have sat for more than 20,000 hours during that time.

LACK OF EXERCISE

This lack of movement because of prolonged sitting does not stop once we leave school. I have asked thousands of people from all walks of life, 'What is the total number of hours you spend sitting down during an average day?' Answers ranged from four to a staggering 14 hours, the average being over 10 hours a day, which is nearly two-thirds of our waking life.

It is because many of us use so few of our muscles to their maximum capacity that we slowly begin to lose much of our flexibility, until we end up in old age scarcely able to move. Yet even at the age of 85, Alexander could balance perfectly on one leg while he swung the other leg over the back of a chair 1 m (3 ft) high, a feat that most people in their 30s would find difficult.

OUR FEAR REFLEX IS CONSTANTLY AND INAPPROPRIATELY STIMULATED

Throughout our childhood, and also in adult life, we all have experiences that make us withdraw. These include being reprimanded by parents, teachers and employers, being ridiculed by our peer group, and being rejected by our friends and loved ones. These incidents, if frequently repeated, can cause us to become excessively introverted and we will eventually adopt a posture that reflects our defensive attitude. This posture will remain long after the initial cause has ceased. A defensive posture – hunched or rounded shoulders, a collapsed torso and excessive tension in the neck muscles – is easy to identify.

THE SPEED WITH WHICH WE OFTEN HAVE TO ACCOMPLISH OUR TASKS

We often have to accomplish many of our activities in a set time, far more than previous generations did. This will certainly lead to anxiety and tension and, if constantly repeated, will cause us to adopt certain postures in response.

THE GOAL-ORIENTED ATTITUDE THAT WE ARE TAUGHT AS CHILDREN AND AT WORK

Alexander talked at length on the subject of 'goal orientation'. He referred to civilized man as a race of end-gainers. What he meant by this was that we are often more interested in achieving an end than experiencing the means whereby we reach that end. Because of this, our posture and co-ordination can be severely affected in the process of performing even the simplest tasks. It is almost unbelievable how much tremendous force intelligent human beings can employ throughout their whole bodies while performing such a simple action as standing up, just because they are more interested in the end result than in how they should perform such an activity. If unchecked, this will cause postural difficulties in later life.

A DISTINCT LACK OF INTEREST IN THE PRESENT

A lack of interest in the present is mainly brought on by the habitual way in which we are constantly looking to the future. We are encouraged by society always to want more, always to look to the future which promises to be even more fulfilling. For example, for months and months before Christmas we are bombarded with advertisements for Christmas, and then on Christmas Day itself, enticements for the summer holidays begin.

THE DEVELOPMENT OF HABITS, BOTH PHYSICAL AND MENTAL

We all form habits, both of body and mind, most of which are below our level of consciousness. These habits feel comfortable to us and are therefore difficult to change since new ways of being can feel strange to begin with. These habits, however, can often put our whole organism out of balance and we may soon start to resume rigid positions and become fixed in one posture or another.

Posture is an ever-changing process, depending on where we are in space. It could be said that 'bad posture' is a posture that is fixed in one place and that 'good posture' is a posture that is always varying with different moods and movements of the body. The possible effects of a rigid posture can be:

Shallow breathing

This will, of course, affect the whole system as oxygen is needed by every organ in the body.

Over-tiredness

The constant effort needed to keep a particular posture drains us of our energy, which could be used to do the things we enjoy.

Stress

Our whole system will be under constant tension, which will eventually develop into pain.

Depression

It is well known that many people who suffer from depression tend to have a very pronounced slumped posture.

THE ORIGINS OF POOR POSTURE

It may be as early as the age of five or six that a child's posture starts to deteriorate, and by the age of nine or 10 the beautiful upright way of being starts to diminish. The child's defensive posture against a hostile world becomes frozen in time and the seeds of future ill health may be already sown. The effects of the long years of bending over a school desk can clearly be seen in many adults in the form of a rounded back or hunched shoulders. Many diseases and common ailments are caused or made worse by the tensions we unconsciously hold within us.

The cost of misusing our bodies is great, not only to ourselves personally, but also to the community. Losses in productivity through back pain alone cost millions each year, for instance. Clearly some serious re-thinking is required but, unfortunately, common sense seems to be lacking in so many areas of our lives. If you arrived home one day to find water dripping through the ceiling, you would not just paper over the wet patch; you would first find the reason for the leak to prevent the problem getting worse. Why is it, then, that when it comes to our health we look only at symptoms and rarely investigate the fundamental causes of so many of our illnesses?

The answer is that we simply do not know where to start, and this is where the Alexander Technique comes in.

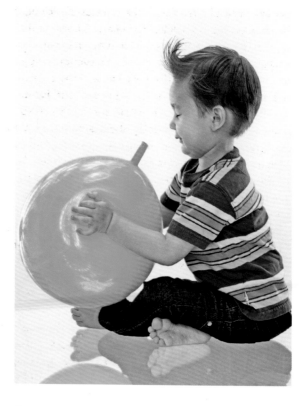

↑ Young children's backs are nearly always straight and aligned without effort.

THE PRESSURES OF EVERYDAY LIVING

In this section I hope to make clear how Alexander's discovery can be of use to us in our everyday lives. As you will remember, his vocal problems stemmed from unnecessary muscle tension which

Note

It is important at this stage to note that better posture is only a by-product of practising the Alexander Technique and not, as many people think, the end in itself. By freeing muscular tension, our whole body has a chance to work more naturally, thus restoring the natural posture and ease of movement we lost in childhood.

occurred when he reacted to the stimulus of reciting. Today we are bombarded with stimuli from all quarters because the world about us moves at such a fast pace. Our automatic reflex system is under constant pressure to keep up with the ever-growing pace of life, and we often do not feel we have time to think before we act. For this reason we start to function in unconscious, habitual ways.

We rarely stop to think whether there may be an easier or more appropriate way of going about even the simplest tasks, and our bodies begin to build up severe tensions, often completely unnoticed until we start to feel pain. A good example of this is the learner driver who clenches the steering wheel with such a strong grip that his hands ache afterwards. He is unaware of this completely unnecessary and inappropriate over-activity of the muscular system. Because of the enormous demands put on us by modern-day living, we build up stress that for the most part goes unnoticed and therefore unchecked.

We have made our lives far more complex than they really need to be. Just consider for a moment how stressful a simple task like shopping has become. We take our car to the shops, drive around for 10 minutes looking for a parking space and then watch in frustration as someone takes the space we have been waiting for. When we eventually find a space, we usually have only limited time to do the shopping so, if anything delays us, we have to rush back to our car before we get a parking ticket. Similarly, think about getting the children to school on time. We have all seen exhausted parents standing outside the school in the morning. Most children have a completely different sense of time from adults, so parents have constantly to nag their children to be punctual, and this is a strain on all concerned.

There are countless situations in everyday life that cause us to be stressed. This stress is then transmitted into muscular tension and, if left unchecked, could go on to contribute to numerous stress-related illnesses, including hypertension, coronary thrombosis, tension headaches, osteoarthritis and back pain. The amount of money spent on drugs to combat illnesses that we are often causing ourselves is enormous.

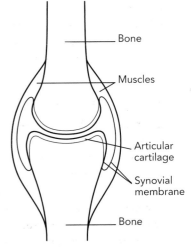

Bone

Muscles

Articular cartilage

Synovial membrane

Bone

↑ Healthy joint.

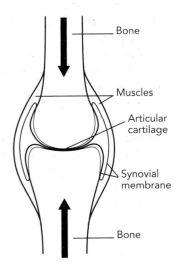

Bone

Muscles

Articular cartilage

Synovial membrane

Bone

↑ Arthritic joint. Over-tensed muscles can cause bones to be pulled together, which can eventually wear the joint out.

Common health problems that can be helped

HYPERTENSION

Hypertension is raised blood pressure, which can rise to a point where there is a risk of cardiac damage or stroke. The cause of high blood pressure is still obscure; at present it is generally believed to occur when the smaller arteries go into spasm. It is thought that this spasm is produced by adrenaline and that adrenaline is produced by emotional, mental or physical strain.

During the 1960s and 1970s, Professor Frank Pierce Jones conducted as series of studies at Tufts University in the United States which used electromyography and EMG equipment to show that the Alexander Technique could produce a marked reduction in stress levels. This is obviously an attractive alternative to the many drugs available because, not only do Alexander lessons produce no adverse side-effects, but they may well be cheaper than many of the expensive hypotensive drugs.

CORONARY THROMBOSIS

Coronary thrombosis, more commonly known as a heart attack, is caused by a narrowing of a major branch of one of the coronary arteries. It could be that this narrowing is caused by the over-tensing of the muscles that surround this particular artery. In his book *The Alexander Principle*, Doctor Wilfred Barlow reports:

I see a good number of people who have had a coronary thrombosis. I have never yet seen a case in which the upper chest was not markedly raised and over-contracted. I regard it as essential that such patients should be taught to release their chest tension and to do so in a way that is accompanied by an improvement in their general use.

GASTRO-INTESTINAL CONDITIONS

Gastro-intestinal conditions figure high on the list of stress-related disorders. An example of this is the stomach ulcer, an extremely painful condition often associated with high-pressure occupations, which subject people to constant undue strain. An ulcer, or a similar ailment, will often develop within a short period as a signal to slow down.

One of the main aims of the Technique is to help us take our time and, by doing so, accomplish far more – think of the saying, 'More haste, less speed.'

by the Alexander Technique

TENSION HEADACHES

Tension headaches are extremely common today. They are usually caused by over-tightening of the neck and shoulder muscles (the sterno-mastoid and the trapezius). In my experience, Alexander pupils who suffer from headaches say that the pain soon becomes less intense and the headaches less frequent. It is also my experience that, when a pupil comes to me with a headache, once they are able to relax the appropriate muscles, the pain has often gone by the end of the lesson.

MIGRAINE

Many millions of people suffer from this ailment and, while this condition is often related to a hormonal imbalance, many people can be helped by learning to release some of the tension that they hold around the neck, head, shoulders and face. The medical profession states that, although migraines are due to a chemical imbalance, they can be provoked or made worse by stressful conditions such as anxiety, loud noises, physical and mental fatigue, emotional upset and depression.

INSOMNIA

Insomnia is often caused by anxiety in some form. People who suffer from this condition often have an over-active mind – they worry about details of the day and consequently become more annoyed when they cannot sleep. By practising the Alexander Technique they can release much of the tension that has built up over the years and this, in turn, helps them to feel calmer and able to sleep better, thus breaking the cycle.

OSTEOARTHRITIS

Osteoarthritis is the term applied to the chronic degeneration and ultimate deformity of the bones that make up a joint. This could be caused by a permanent over-tightening of the muscles that connect the two bones involved.

As you can see from the illustration on page 39 (bottom), the muscles shorten to such an extent that the two connecting bones start to rub against each other and begin to wear down. Just imagine how much tension it takes to erode a substance as hard as bone. It is important to note, however, that once the muscle is able to lengthen again, the bones return to their original position (as in the illustration at the top of page 39) and, because bone is living tissue, it could repair itself again. Thus arthritis sufferers can experience relief once they begin to become aware of, and to release, the muscle tension they have unconsciously been holding.

ASTHMA

Asthma is a common chronic inflammatory disease of the airways and has recurring symptoms, such as airflow obstruction and constriction of the muscles in the walls of the bronchioles. Symptoms include wheezing, cough, chest tightness, and shortness of breath. By releasing tension, asthma sufferers can learn how to breathe in a different way and many people I have taught have lessened or eradicated the effects of asthma and other breathing problems. In fact Alexander himself had breathing problems that he cured himself of while developing his Technique. (See Chapter 13.)

BACK PAIN

Back pain is one of the most common illnesses in our society today. In the UK, 11 billion working days are lost annually because of back pain and about 85 per cent of all American adults suffer back pain at some point in their lives. Because so many people are affected by back pain, I have dedicated a whole chapter to the subject (see Chapter 12).

Most of the problems in our life stem from the simple fact that we are very rarely totally present while we perform our tasks; we are usually thinking about something else completely. Alexander called this 'the mind-wandering habit'. It is impossible to put the Technique into practice until we become attentive to each action we perform. As the growing pressures of living in the 21st century place ever-increasing demands on our bodies and minds, it might be worth remembering this saying, 'Whoever wins the rat race will still be a rat at the end of it!'

PREVENTING ILLNESS

It is important to mention that, although most people do not turn to the Alexander Technique until they are in pain, a healthy person can benefit enormously from it. Not only will it result in a lightness of being and increased awareness, but will help to prevent many of the problems already mentioned. With the growing pressures around us, it is essential to find a practical way of being aware of, and thus able to let go of, the many tensions we accumulate from day to day.

Reducing stress

It is obvious that most of us cannot change our lifestyles. The children still have to be taken to school on time, the bills still have to be paid and we still need to perform tasks that are potentially stressful. However, we can choose not to react to the ever-present stimuli in a way that is detrimental to our wellbeing. You can start to do this by practising the following:

Give yourself plenty of time to get where you are going. Try not to leave things until the last minute, especially when being late is bound to cause tension.

Avoid deadlines whenever possible. Don't tie yourself down to specific times when more general ones will do. For example, say 'I will meet you between 8.30 and 9.00' rather than 'I will see you at 8.45'. Try to remember that life is not an emergency!

Allow time for yourself. Don't run yourself down. Set aside some time each day for the things you really enjoy doing. Try to listen to your body, as there are many signs our body gives us before illness occurs. It is worth remembering: 'Human beings say that time passes away. But time says that it is the human beings that pass away.'

Live each day to the full. Concern yourself with the present; yesterday cannot be changed and tomorrow has not yet come. Remember that the only time we ever have is today. Thomas Carlyle once wrote: 'Our main business is not to see what lies dimly at a distance, but to do what lies clearly at hand.'

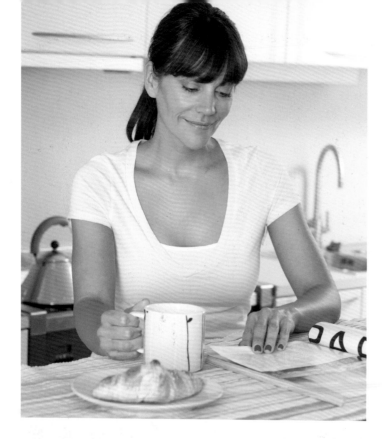

← Taking your time while eating and drinking can dramatically reduce stress.

exercise

STOP AND DO NOTHING

1 The first thing to do to reduce muscle tension is to stop and do nothing for at least a few minutes each day, just to be with yourself. In this way you can begin to notice tension or muscular strain before it builds up and causes further physical problems. Find just 10 minutes in your day to go off and be alone – it does not matter whether you sit or lie down. For this short time it is best not to have the radio or television on and to avoid any other distractions.

2 Just practise being alone with your thoughts. In this way you can begin to become aware of the excessive muscular tensions throughout your body. At first the 10 minutes will feel endless, but as you get used to this quiet space in your day the 10 minutes will pass in no time at all.

3 It is hard to put aside all your responsibilities at first, but they will all be taken care of in due course – we forget that to take care of ourselves is one of our most important responsibilities which is often neglected.

Pat's story

Pat Vince
Age: 58 | Occupation: bank clerk

When Pat started Alexander lessons she had osteoarthritis of the neck and spin and had raised blood pressure. She had tried everything, including osteopaths, chiropractors, physiotherapy, traction and painkillers. She had this to say about her experience of the Technique:

'I knew absolutely nothing about the Alexander Technique and viewed it with a certain amount of scepticism. I did not hope for very much when I began my lessons, because of past experiences. My main aim was for some relief to the back pain that I had had for many years but I was not too optimistic. I was also interested in the possible help for tension, worry and high blood pressure.

Now nearly a year later, attending one class a week and one weekend workshop, and no private lessons, I have been transformed by the Technique. I have found great relief from back pain, my tension and worry are very much reduced and my doctor has given up even taking my blood pressure.

I have become much more aware of the workings of my body and have begun to use it in a way that is much more economical. I become aware when parts of my body become tense and I know now how to 'relax' them, and when my body is saying that it has had enough I am able to leave things till tomorrow instead of insisting that they have to be done today. The lessons on the causes and remedies of worry were most beneficial and the psychology of using your mind in order to create a change in the body helped to reduce the constant tensions in my mind, with the result that I am a much less tense person and a lot of my worries have just vanished.

I realize that I have much more to learn, but I am more than happy with the benefits that I have received so far.'

There are an increasing number of stress-management courses and relaxation classes available, yet many of us hardly ever get to the root of what makes us stressed in the first place. In the Western world, we have insurance policies to protect us from the external changes that may happen in our lives, yet we rarely consider protecting ourselves from the internal changes that result in so many ailments.

It is interesting that, many years ago, people in China paid their doctor only when they were well and not, as we do today, when they fell sick. As a result, there was a great incentive for the doctor to keep his patients well. We often fail to value our health until we become ill, so we ignore the signals our body is giving us. We do not realize that stiffness and inflexibility can nearly always be avoided if we use ourselves in a different way. The Alexander Technique helps to free us from the habits of a lifetime, bringing renewed flexibility and ease of movement.

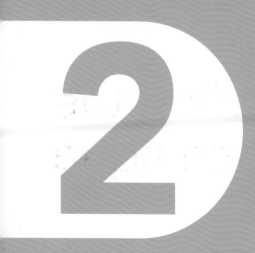

Understanding the Alexander Technique

4

Inhibition

Between stimulus and response, there is a space.
In that space lies our freedom and power to choose our response.
In our response lies our growth and our happiness.

VIKTOR FRANKL, *MAN'S SEARCH FOR MEANING*

Inhibition is perhaps the most important of all the principles of the Alexander Technique. Inhibition is simply the opposite of volition. It is a moment of withholding consent to an automatic reaction or habit. The word 'inhibition' has been commonly used to describe a self-imposed suppression of behaviour or emotions ever since Sigmund Freud used the term in this way in his writings on psychoanalysis. This is not, however, how Alexander used the word; there is no suppressing, just creating a space in which to think. The dictionary definition of 'inhibition', however, is: 'The restraint of direct expression of an instinct'.

Alexander realized that in order to bring about a desirable change in the use of his body he would first have to inhibit (or stop) his habitual, instinctive responses to a given stimulus.

By pausing for a moment before an action takes place, we have time to use our reasoning powers to choose which is the most efficient and appropriate way of performing such an action. This vital step of creating a space between the stimulus and response can lead us toward having the power to choose freely on every level.

Before the brain can be used as an instrument for action, it has to be used as an instrument for inaction. The ability to delay (pause) our responses until we are adequately prepared is what is meant by inhibition. This moment of pausing before acting has nothing to do with freezing or suppression, neither is it about performing actions slowly.

INSTINCTIVE INHIBITION

One of the best examples of natural and instinctive inhibition is the cat. You can observe this even in a domestic cat, when it first sees a mouse. It does not immediately rush and capture its prey, but waits until the appropriate moment in order to achieve the highest chance of success.

It is an interesting fact that, while cats are fine examples of inhibition and control, they are at the same time among the fastest creatures on earth. The cat's ability to pause is instinctual; in other words, it is an automatic function of the subconscious brain. Man, by contrast, has this potential subject to conscious control, and it is this difference which defines a clear line between man and the animal world.

Alexander firmly believed that we have to delay our instantaneous response to the many stimuli that bombard us each

A cat inhibits the desire to spring prematurely, and controls to a deliberate end its eagerness for the instant gratification of a natural appetite.
FREDERICK MATTHIAS ALEXANDER

exercise

DON'T REACT IMMEDIATELY

1 Every time the telephone or the doorbell rings, pause for just two seconds before answering. You may find this simple exercise harder to do than it first seems.

2 Whenever you find yourself in a heated discussion or an argument, try counting backwards from 10 to one before responding. As well as being a useful exercise in inhibition it will give you time to think about what you really want to convey.

3 Choose a simple activity, such as cleaning your teeth or doing the washing-up, and occasionally stop completely for a moment or two and be aware of any excess tension you may be holding in your body. You may even be able to see it in the mirror. If you do this each day for several days running, you are likely to find that the areas of tension will be the same each day. Being aware of the tension is the first step in being able to change the habit.

4 Place a chair in front of a mirror. Stand up and sit down in your normal way and see if you can notice any habitual tendencies (i.e. any one thing that occurs every time), but do not worry if you can't. Repeat, but this time pause for a moment or two before carrying out the action, while you consciously refuse to sit down or stand up in your normal way. Soon you will see that there are many different ways of performing the same action. See whether you notice any differences between the first and second way of performing the action. (You may see a difference in the mirror or you may feel a difference on a sensory level.)

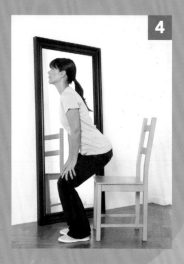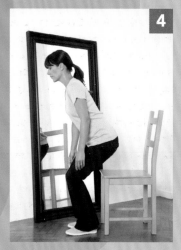

day, if we are to cope with our rapidly changing environment. As our direct dependence on the body for subsistence has decreased, our instinct has become increasingly unreliable so that it is now necessary, through the use of inhibition, to employ our conscious powers to replace these outmoded instincts.

CONSCIOUS INHIBITION

If we are ever to change our habitual responses to given stimuli we have to make a conscious decision to refuse to act in our old automatic and unconscious patterns; that is, to say 'no' to our ingrained habits of use.

By inhibiting our initial instinctive action we have the choice to make an entirely different decision. Inhibition is an essential and integral step when practising the Technique, and Alexander summarized it thus:

> Boiled down it all comes to inhibiting a particular reaction to a given stimulus – but no one will see it that way. They will see it as getting in and out of a chair the right way. It is nothing of the kind. It is that a pupil decides what he will, or will not, consent to do.

There are many old sayings and proverbs that point to the wisdom of thought before action, including: 'Think on the end before you begin', 'Look before you leap' and 'Good and quickly seldom meet'.

If you are able to prevent yourself from performing your habitual actions then you are half-way to your goal. To refrain from an action is as much an act as actually performing an activity, because in both cases the nervous system is employed. It is also possible, and indeed desirable, to inhibit any unwanted habits and tendencies, not only before an action takes place, but also during any given activity. The exercises on pages 52 and 54 will help you to see what it feels like when you do not react immediately to certain stimuli.

You may need to carry out the above exercises a few times before you are aware of certain patterns of behaviour.

One of the most noticeable tendencies that Alexander observed in himself was that he constantly tightened his neck muscles. Initially, he presumed that this phenomenon was merely a personal idiosyncrasy, but later observations showed him that this

exercise

NECK TENSION

To demonstrate that the head is pulled back by excess tension of the neck muscles during a movement, follow these steps:

1 Sit in a chair.

2 Place your left hand on the left side of the neck, and the right hand on the right side of the neck, so that the two middle fingers are just touching each other at the back of the neck (at the base of the skull).

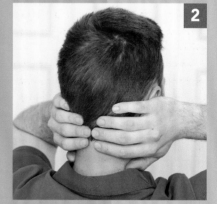

3 Stand up.

4 Then sit down again.

5 By being aware of the pressure on your fingers, while you are sitting down or standing up, you will be able to detect any pulling back of the head. Watch for a feeling that the head is being pressed back into the hands. This indicates neck tension and the head being pulled back.

6 Perform the exercise several times, as you may well notice more tension on the second or third repetition.

was not the case at all – this tensing up of the neck muscles was practically universal.

This habit invariably leads to a pulling back of the head on to the spine, thus compressing the intervertebral discs and shortening the structure. This constant downward pressure on the spine may well be one of the reasons why most people 'shrink' with age. The pulling back of the head also interferes dramatically with what Alexander called the Primary Control. As mentioned earlier (see page 25), this is a term for a system of reflexes which takes place in the neck area and has the power to control all the other reflexes to direct the body in a co-ordinated and balanced way. It is called 'primary' because, if this reflex action is interfered with, all the other muscles throughout the body can be affected.

If we are truly pulling our heads back habitually and interfering with the Primary Control, then the implications are very serious. Our co-ordination and balance can be severely affected and we will be forced to hold ourselves in a rigid fashion to stop ourselves from falling over. In other words, when we come to move we will actually be working against ourselves.

A learner driver who grips the steering wheel too tightly with one hand may have difficulty moving the steering wheel with the other. As a driving instructor, I encountered many people who thought there was something wrong with the steering mechanism because the wheel would not move very easily! They were of course totally oblivious to the tension in their hands, arms and shoulders.

EXPERIMENTAL EVIDENCE

In the mid-1920s, Rudolf Magnus, a professor of pharmacology at the University of Utrecht, became interested in exploring the role our physiological mechanisms play in affecting our movement and wellbeing. Magnus was struck by the central function of the reflexes that governed the position of an animal's head in relation to the rest of its body and to its environment. With his colleagues, he performed a series of experiments to establish the nature and function of postural reflexes throughout the body. He wrote over 300 papers on the subject, pointing to the fact that it was the head-neck reflexes that were the central controlling mechanism responsible for orienting the animal to his environment, both in assuming a posture for a particular purpose and also in restoring the animal to a resting posture after an action.

Magnus's experiments confirmed what Alexander had discovered in himself a quarter of a century earlier: that in all animals the mechanism of the body is set up in such a way that the head leads a movement and then the body follows. In retrospect, this seems to be an obvious statement because all the senses are in the head and, if we follow our senses as we are designed to do, then our head will automatically lead the way. This phenomenon occurs naturally in all animals with the exception of humans, in whom it can clearly be seen that the head is constantly being thrown back when a movement takes place.

The other major discovery made by Magnus was what he called 'the righting reflex'. He noticed that, after an action which requires extra tension has taken place (for example, a cat leaping onto a table), a set of 'righting reflexes' come into play that restore the animal (or human) to its normal composed posture. The relationship of the head, neck and back is an essential factor when this righting mechanism is in operation. Therefore, it is true to say that, when a person stiffens the neck muscles and pulls their head back and down, not only is the body's natural co-ordination impeded, but the body is also prevented from returning to its natural state of ease and equilibrium.

What a piece of work is a man! How noble in reason, how infinite in faculty, in form and moving how express and admiral, in action how like an angel, in apprehension how like a god – the beauty of the world, the paragon of animals!

WILLIAM SHAKESPEARE, *HAMLET*

exercise

HOW DO YOUR ARMS FEEL?

1 Another exercise to try is to stand with both arms resting by your sides. Take a moment to be aware of what they feel like. Do they feel the same or does one arm feel longer, heavier, freer, than the other?

2 Without thinking, raise one arm up to the side so that it is level with your shoulder. Hold it there for a moment or two and then relax the arm back down to the side. Do the same action again with the other arm, but first inhibit your action for a few seconds so that you can be aware in more detail of raising the arm up the second time.

3 Notice if you can feel any difference between arms after you have performed this exercise. People often experience a feeling of lightness in the arm when they paused before the movement. Repeat the same exercise, but this time reverse the process, pausing before raising the first arm.

Alexander once commented on this quoted passage, saying:

> These words seem to me now to be contradicted by what I
> have discovered in myself and others. For what could be less
> 'noble in reason', less 'infinite in faculty' than that man,
> despite his potentialities, should have fallen into such error
> in the use of himself, and in this way brought about such a
> lowering in his standard of functioning that in everything he
> attempts to accomplish, these harmful conditions tend to
> become more and more exaggerated? In consequence, how
> many people are there today of whom it may be said, as
> regards their use of themselves, 'in form and moving how
> express and admirable'? Can we any longer consider man in
> this regard 'the paragon of animals'?

Yet if we are able to inhibit this unconscious habit of tensing up our
neck muscles, then this will free our whole body to perform actions
in such a way that they become as much a joy to watch as they are
to carry out.

Jacob Bronowski saw inhibition as such a crucial ability to the
whole of the human race that he wrote the following in his famous
book *The Ascent of Man*:

> We are nature's unique experiment to make the rational
> intelligence prove sounder than the reflex. Success or failure
> of this experiment depends on the basic human ability to
> impose a delay between the stimulus and the response.

5

Directions

The Alexander Technique gives us all the things we have been looking for in a system of physical education; relief from strain due to maladjustment and consequent improvement in physical and mental health; and along with this a heightening of consciousness on all levels. We cannot ask more from any system; nor, if we seriously desire to alter human beings in a desirable direction, can we ask any less.

ALDOUS HUXLEY, *MEANS AND ENDS*

During Alexander's years of experimentation, he was led to a long consideration of directing his body. He had to admit that he had never once given any thought to how he directed himself in activity. He had used himself habitually in the way that felt 'natural' and 'right' to him. Having effectively prevented his unconscious stereotyped patterns from repeating themselves, and having made a space between stimulus and response, Alexander then brought his brain into action by formulating conscious verbal instructions and sending them to the part of the body which he had been unable to control before.

In his book *The Use of the Self*, Alexander described 'giving directions' as:

> A process which involves projecting messages from the brain to the body's mechanisms and conducting the energy necessary for the use of these mechanisms.

It is possible to direct *specific* parts of yourself (for example, you can think of your fingers lengthening) or to direct your *whole* self (such as when thinking of your entire structure lengthening). You can also direct yourself through space by consciously deciding where you are going and how you intend to get there. It is important to realize that giving these 'directions' is an actual experience, and you will need some Alexander lessons to learn how to give them. It is nearly impossible to give these directions without the experience of specific quality of muscle tone which a trained teacher can impart.

THE PRIMARY DIRECTION

Alexander realized that the root cause of many problems was that the over-tightening of the neck muscles caused an interference with the Primary Control which, in turn, threw the whole body out of balance. He realized that the first and most important step was to give the necessary directions to ensure a lessening of tension in the neck area, restoring the normal functioning of the Primary Control.

The main direction he devised was:

> *Allow the neck to be free*
> in such a way that
> *The head can go forward and upward*
> in order that
> *The back can lengthen and widen.*

There are many slight variations of these orders:

'Allow the neck to be free' is sometimes changed to:
> 'Let the neck be free'
> 'Think of the neck as being free'
> 'Think of the neck muscles releasing'
> 'Think of not stiffening the neck'
> 'Relax the neck'. (Alexander himself initially used this order, but he changed the wording when he found that his pupils tended to over-relax their neck muscles.)

'The head can go forward and upward' is often changed to:
> 'Think of allowing the head going forward and up'
> 'Let the head go forward and up'
> 'Allow the head to go forward and upward'
> 'Think of not pulling the head backward and downward'.

'The back can lengthen and widen' can also become:
> 'Think of the back lengthening and widening'
> 'Allow the back to lengthen and widen'
> 'Think of not shortening and narrowing the back'
> 'Let the entire body expand in space'.

ALLOW THE NECK TO BE FREE

This instruction should eliminate the excess tension that is almost always present in the muscles of the neck. This is essential if the head is ever going to move freely on the spine, in order for the Primary Control to perform its natural function. This should always be the first direction given because, unless the Primary Control is able to organize the rest of the body, any other directions will be relatively ineffective.

I have found it very useful to give actual images to my pupils. Many people find that thinking of the head being like a balloon filled with helium and floating upward is very helpful. Others find thinking of the head as finely balanced, like a ping-pong ball on top of a fountain, also very useful.

It is also important to realize what Alexander meant when he referred to the neck. I personally do not think of this as neck muscles or the vertebrae in the neck. Although Alexander never actually said where the neck was, he always indicated that it was high up away from the shoulders and situated between the ears.

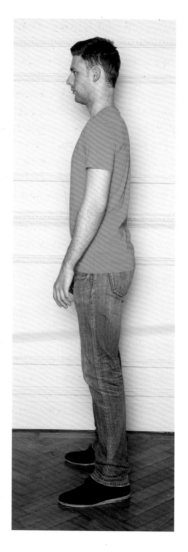

↑ Thinking of the neck as being free and allowing the head to go forward and up can help to bring the body into balance.

ALLOW THE HEAD TO GO FORWARD AND UPWARD

This tells you in which way the neck needs to be free. If you just thought of your neck being free without any qualifying instructions, your head might well fall forward and down. This direction helps you to keep the head balanced in such a way that, when the neck muscles are released, the head goes slightly forward; this keeps the body poised or can take the whole body into movement, allowing the mechanisms of the body to function naturally and freely.

If you think only of the head going forward and not upward, it would invariably drop downward, causing increased muscular tension in the neck area. It is important to realize that the forward direction is the head going forward *on the spine* (as if you are about to nod your head affirmatively). The upward direction of the head is *away from the spine* and not away from the Earth, although these may well be the same when the structure is upright (see the illustration, right).

Centre of gravity of the head

Upward direction of the head

Pivot point where the head is balanced on the spine

Forward direction of the head

Lengthening of the spine

⬆ Diagram of the head showing the directions of head movement.

ALLOW THE BACK TO LENGTHEN AND WIDEN

Since it is the spine that shortens because of excess muscular tension when the head is pulled back, this direction will encourage a lengthening of the whole structure. In fact, many people who practise the Alexander Technique actually increase in height by 2.5 cm (1 in) or more! The reason a widening direction is included is that it is easy for a narrowing to occur while the lengthening process is taking place.

These three primary directions are in themselves very simple and straightforward. However, because of our 'debauched kinaesthesia' (meaning a distorted sense of where your body is in space, this was a favourite term of Alexander's, which can be used to impress people at parties!), they can be confusing when first practised. This is partly because they are so simple and we are used to thinking in a more complicated way. It is hard for us to believe that the solution to what may have been a longstanding problem can indeed be so simple. We live in a fast-moving world and, when results do not happen immediately, we presume that we are doing something wrong. Be patient and observant and realize that changing the habits of a lifetime does take time.

It is strongly advised that when you start giving directions you have at least a few lessons from a trained Alexander teacher to make sure you are on the right track.

Note

It is important to realize that you will probably need some Alexander lessons to experience the directions described in this chapter. It is very easy to start to 'do' the directions instead of merely thinking of them. To 'do' the directions is for Alexander called 'end gaining' (see page 101), and this will be of no value to you at all. In fact, it may well be counter-productive.

SECONDARY DIRECTIONS

There are many secondary directions – too many to detail. Whereas the main or primary directions can be applied universally, the secondary directions may be applied to certain conditions or ailments. For example, if a person comes to me suffering from rounded shoulders I may give them an instruction to, 'Think of your shoulders going away from each other' or, if someone comes to me with arthritic fingers, I may ask them to, 'Think of your fingers lengthening'.

Some people just think or repeat the words to themselves, while others have a three-dimensional image in their head. At the end of the day, use whatever is best for you.

On page 61 are some examples of secondary directions commonly used in the teaching of the Technique.

There are many more directions to suit an individual's needs, but the primary directions *always* precede any secondary direction that may be given.

The words 'think of' may often be substituted by the word 'allow' or 'think of allowing' or 'let', depending on the teacher's or pupil's preference. It can be interesting to see if they have different effects on the body. The most important thing to remember at all times is to bring about a change by thinking alone, and not to try to 'do' anything to bring about a change. As I have said previously, when you try to *do* anything it always increases the muscular tension, which is the very opposite of what you are trying to achieve.

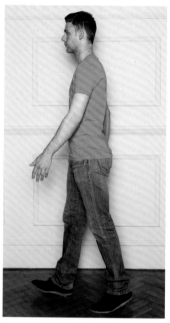

↑ Many people do not bend their knees when walking. Thinking of the knees moving forward and away from each other can help to make walking easier and more fluid.

exercise

THE HEAD LEADING THE BODY

1 Look at an object of your choice.

2 Without taking your eyes off the object, allow them to get closer and closer to the object.

3 As the head begins to move toward the object, let the rest of the body follow. This will show you how the head can lead the body.

It is important to make sure that you are not tensing your neck muscles and pulling your head backward, otherwise it will be only your head that will be getting closer without the body necessarily following.

exercise

IMAGINARY BALLOONS

Try this one on yourself and then on a friend.

1 The actual weight of an arm is approximately 3.6 kg (8 lb) – equivalent to four bags of sugar. So, with this in mind, begin to raise your arms up slowly to the sides.

2 It should take you about half a minute to raise your arms up until they are horizontal. Keep thinking of the actual weight of your arms.

3 Hold your arms at the horizontal position for another half a minute or so to get a sense of how heavy they really are.

4 Slowly lower your arms back down to your sides.

5 Take a minute or two and make a note (either mental or on paper) of how your arms feel.

6 Wait for your arms to feel normal again, moving them a little if necessary.

7 Now let your arms hang down by your sides and imagine a balloon being placed between your arm and rib-cage on each side.

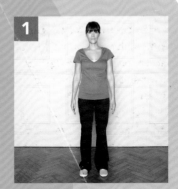

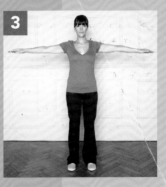

8 Imagine the two balloons being slowly blown up, simultaneously.

9 As the balloons are being blown up they will gently push your arms up.

10 When your arms are level with your shoulders, imagine your arms being gently supported by the balloons.

11 Now imagine the air being slowly let out of the balloons so that your arms descend gradually down to your sides.

12 Make a note of how your arms feel now. Note whether they feel any different from before. If they do, you have proved that thought actually does affect functioning because you have performed exactly the same action in each case.

6

Faulty Sensory Appreciation

Everyone wants to be right, but no one stops to consider if their idea of right is right.

FREDERICK MATTHIAS ALEXANDER

The main difficulty people have when starting to practise the Alexander Technique is the very difficulty experienced by Alexander himself – namely, that they are suffering from an unreliable sensory appreciation of themselves. This simply means that their proprioception (their sense of position) and their kinaesthesia (their sense of movement) have both become faulty and are actually giving false information as to where they are in space and what they are doing at any given time. As I have already mentioned, Marjorie Barlow, Alexander teacher and Alexander's niece, often told her pupils: 'Just make sure you know what you are doing and make sure you can stop doing it if you still want to.'

Because many of us suffer from a faulty sensory mechanism, we often do not have any idea of what we are doing. We may be standing or sitting leaning backward and think we are standing or sitting perfectly straight.

A good example of Faulty Sensory Appreciation sometimes happens when we go to the hairdresser. You may have had the experience of the hairdresser asking you to put your head straight, so that he or she can cut your hair evenly, and then moving your head after you have done so. This is because, although you think that your head is straight, it is actually inclined to one side. Alexander put it this way:

> There must be, in the first place, a clear realization by the pupil that he suffers from a defect or defects needing eradication. In the second place, the teacher must make a lucid diagnosis of such defects and decide upon the means of dealing with them. He (the pupil) acknowledges that he suffers from mental delusions regarding his physical acts and that his sensory appreciation, or kinaesthesis, is defective and misleading. In other words, he realizes that his sense register of the amount of muscular tension needed to accomplish even a simple act of everyday life is faulty and harmful, and his mental conception of such conditions as relaxation and concentration is impossible in practical application.
>
> For there can be no doubt that man on the subconscious plane now relies too much on a debauched sense of feeling or of sense-appreciation for the guidance of his psychophysical mechanism, and that he is gradually becoming more and more overbalanced emotionally, with very harmful and far-reaching results.

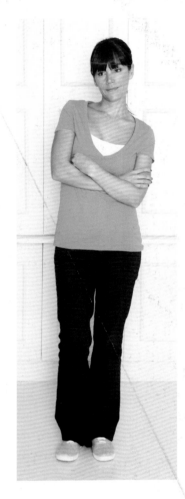

↑ Many people do not feel unbalanced, but it becomes obvious when they see themselves in a mirror.

To simplify this: what we are actually doing and what we think we are doing may be two totally different things.

FOOT POSITION

To demonstrate the above:

1 Without looking at your feet, place them 30 cm (12 in) apart, pointing them straight ahead so that they are parallel to each other.

2 Now look at your feet to see if the intended position of your feet matches the real position.

3 This time look at your feet and place them 23 cm (9 in) apart so that they are parallel.

4 What do they feel like?

Try this exercise on as many people as possible, noticing that the position of the feet can vary enormously from person to person. Then try another exercise:

BACK STRAIGHT

1 Ask a friend to sit on a chair.

2 Place your hand on the lumbar arch of the spine.

3 Ask your friend to sit up straight.

4 Observe how they arch their back by shortening the spine, therefore becoming concave in shape instead of straight.

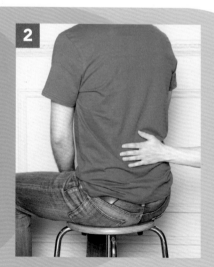

THE KINAESTHETIC SENSE

The kinaesthetic sense is a term mentioned time and time again in connection with the Alexander Technique. The kinaesthetic sense largely uses feedback mechanisms within the muscles themselves which send messages to the brain whenever there is movement of the joints and muscles. These sensations send impulses along nerves to the brain and thus inform it of any movement that takes place, even the movement of the breath. It is extremely important for co-ordination, balance and overall posture.

THE SENSE OF PROPRIOCEPTION

Kinaesthesia and the sense of proprioception are often used interchangeably. Proprioception is the *sense* of the relative position of parts of the body. As with the kinaesthetic sense, it is an internal sense as it is stimulated from within the body itself. This is done via numerous sensory receptors in internal organs and muscles, such as stretch receptors, that are neurologically linked to the brain, which is mainly responsible for the operation of this sense.

As both the sense of proprioception and the kinaesthetic sense rely on feedback from the muscular system, it follows that excessive muscular tension may well interfere with either one or both of these senses. This could distort the information that is given by the body's feedback mechanisms. So the main reasons for our Faulty Sensory Appreciation is probably that many of us hold our

exercise

USING YOUR KINAESTHETIC SENSE

To understand in a practical way what the kinaesthetic sense is:

1 Close your eyes.

2 Slowly raise your left arm out to the side.

3 Without opening your eyes, see if you can feel where your arm is in space.

4 If you have been able to locate the position of your arm without looking, then you must have used your kinaesthetic sense to do so.

body with excessive tension and the strongly contracted muscles grossly interfere with the information that the senses are picking up from the receptors in the joints and muscles. This in turn will affect our sense of proprioception and kinaesthesia. By releasing the tension through the Alexander Technique, we can radically help to reduce these interferences.

If, as Alexander discovered, this sense is supplying us with false information, then the implications are very serious. We may be going about all our daily activities and performing strenuous exercises thinking we are doing one thing when we may be doing exactly the opposite. One of the most common examples of Faulty Sensory Appreciation occurs when teaching is the pupil's inability to tell correctly whether they are upright when standing. Many people think they are upright when in fact they are leaning backward by as much as 20 degrees. In group situations this is particularly noticeable because everyone else can see clearly that a subject is leaning backward, yet they are convinced they are not.

This belief system is so entrenched that when I have guided people into an upright position they actually feel they are leaning forward, so much so that they tense up because they think they are about to fall over. Since many people spend most of their waking hours completely out of balance, their muscles are constantly under strain.

RIGHTS AND WRONGS

In order to make the necessary changes in ourselves, to bring about a new and improved way of moving, we need to do the very thing that feels wrong. Alexander once said:

> The right thing to do would be the last thing we should do, left to ourselves, because it would be the last thing we should think it would be the right thing to do. Everyone wants to be right, but no one stops to consider if their idea of right is right. When people are wrong, the thing that is right is bound to be wrong to them.

So the problem is, in fact, quite complex. It is human nature to move, sit or stand in a way that feels most comfortable. We would not dream of moving in a way that feels strange or even alien to us, and yet this is exactly what is required. As you will remember,

Alexander stumbled across this discovery only because he was using a mirror. He became disheartened when he realized he was doing exactly the opposite of what he had intended to do; that he was trying to put his head forward and up, when in reality he was pulling his head back and down in an even more pronounced way than before.

Alexander used to advise his pupils to 'try and feel wrong', because in that way the pupil would have some small chance of doing the right action. For this reason it is highly recommended initially to take a course of lessons, because it is so easy to increase muscular tension and aggravate any problem (or potential problem) that you have. Because the Alexander teacher has been highly trained and is an objective observer, they can easily detect any extra tension that may occur when you are trying to put something right. They can also impart an experience of lightness and ease of movement which can be used as a point of reference when experimenting with your own movements.

We are conditioned from an early age to be right. We get rewards when we are right and punishments when we are wrong and, like Pavlov's dogs, we begin to form fixed ideas about what is right and wrong and what is good and bad. As we grow up, we form ideas based on what is taught to us at school and by our parents and are often discouraged from thinking for ourselves. Look at

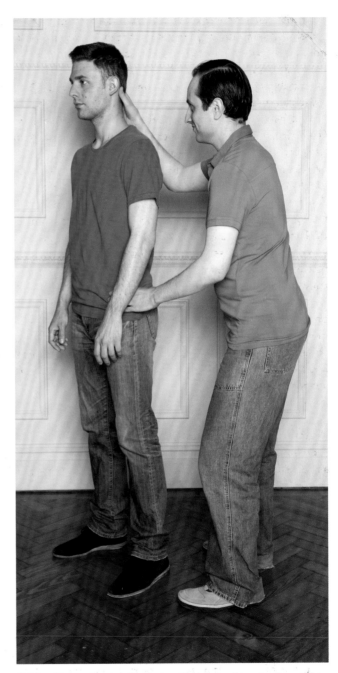

↑ The Alexander teacher helps the student to stand upright without tension.

history. There was a time when the people of Europe 'knew' that the world was flat. They were so convinced of this that anyone who said otherwise and threatened their belief system was ridiculed and often called insane. It was not until Christopher Columbus had sailed right around the world that people would admit they were wrong. In the same way, we walk around with many incorrect concepts about ourselves and would challenge anyone to tell us otherwise!

It is important to have an open mind and a good sense of humour when trying to find your way through this maze of illusions and realities. A pupil will often come to a point of confusion when they begin to realize that their ideas of what they thought to be true were actually based on a false premise. However, this confusion is soon replaced by realization after realization of what is true and what is not. It might be worth thinking about the following sentence from *Illusions* by Richard Bach: 'There is no such thing as a problem without a gift for you in its hands.'

To give some further examples of faulty sensory feelings, try the following exercises:

exercise

RAISING YOUR FINGERS

1 Close your eyes.

2 Raise the index finger of your right hand in front of you so that you feel that it is at eye level and in line with your right ear.

3 Raise the index finger of your left hand so that you feel it is at eye level and in line with your left ear.

4 While keeping your eyes closed, try to line up your fingers so that they are pointing toward each other and are level.

5 Start to move the fingers together and stop when they are nearly touching.

6 Open your eyes and see how close the reality is to your perception.

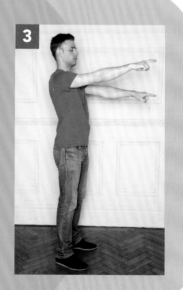

exercise

ARMS UP

1 Ask a friend to stand in front of you with their eyes shut.

2 Ask them to raise their arms so that their arms are level with the shoulders.

3 Check to see (a) if one arm is higher than the other and (b) if both arms are in fact level with the shoulders.

exercise

CLAP YOUR HANDS

1 Close your eyes.

2 Clap your hands so that your hands meet in an even and symmetrical way (i.e. the thumbs and fingers are all touching their counterparts so that their tops are at the same height).

3 Open your eyes to see how close you are.

The implications, and indeed the effects, of Faulty Sensory Appreciation on the human structure can be seen clearly in old age, when many people have become bent or twisted as their body tries to cope with their lack of co-ordination. The only way a pupil can achieve any progress toward making their unreliable sensory feelings more reliable is to accept that, during a course of Alexander lessons, they may well experience ways of moving that initially feel very strange to them. In a comparatively short period of time, however, the new way of being will begin to feel normal and old habits will feel clumsy by comparison.

It is important to point out that the phrase 'unreliable feelings' refers only to sensory feelings and not to emotional feelings. It can be said, however, that the faulty perception of ourselves is bound to affect our physical state which will, in turn, influence our day-to-day emotional condition. Our reason then becomes completely dominated by our emotions to the point where our perception of what is true becomes distorted, thus influencing our ability to discriminate between right and wrong. In this way, a vicious cycle is set up.

exercise

ARE YOU STANDING STRAIGHT?

1 Stand side-on to a mirror and in what you think is an upright posture.

2 Make sure that you are standing as straight as you possibly can. Use the mirror to check whether your feelings of being straight match the reality.

3 If they do not, stand in a posture that you can see is straight, and ask yourself whether you are perceiving yourself in a reliable way.

Be sure to take time over this exercise to observe as much detail as possible. To make this exercise easier, you may like to use two mirrors at an angle to one another. Use a second mirror if you have one, as this can be even more revealing.

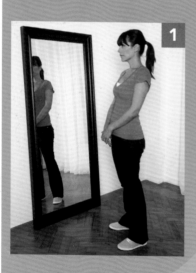
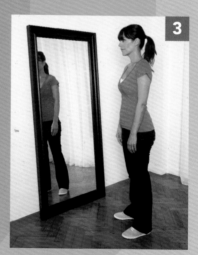

BODY MAPPING

Somewhat related to the subject of Faulty Sensory Appreciation is that of 'body mapping'. A person's body map is their perception, understanding and experience of their own body shape and size, of where their joints move and of how their body functions. Some people have an accurate body map and, as a result, generally move with poise and an easy co-ordination. An inaccurate body map can lead to poor co-ordination or awkward movements.

Body mapping was developed by two American Alexander teachers, William and Barbara Conable. While teaching the Alexander Technique to musicians, they realized that the students were confused about how the body worked and the actual position of certain joints. The Conables saw that by having a clearer idea about the way the body's mechanisms function we can learn to let go of certain habits more quickly. In her book *How to Learn the Alexander Technique*, Barbara Conable sets out many different body mapping errors. I would like to show you some of the most common ones.

Head-spine joint

Many people incorrectly map this joint. When asked to locate the position of this joint they often indicate that it is at the back of the head or even at the top of their shoulders. The joint is approximately between the ears. It is very important to know this when thinking of the neck being free. What Alexander meant by the neck is really the atlanto-occipital joint, as well as the neck muscles themselves, so if you are this mapping this joint incorrectly, it will be much harder, or even impossible, to obtain a free neck.

Arm-body joint

When we look in the mirror we see our arms dangling from our shoulders. Therefore we presume that the bones of the arm are connected to the top of the shoulder. In reality, however, the bones of the arm continue under the skin and muscle. The upper arm (humerus) is connected to the shoulder blade (scapula) which, in turn, is connected to the collar bone (clavicle). It is where the collar bone meets the breast bone (sternum) that the arm really joins to the body. The arms are in effect only 2–5 cm (1–2 in) away from each other.

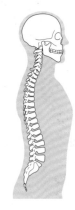

↑ The top of the spine is located at the place between the ears.

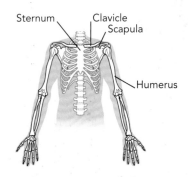

Sternum   Clavicle   Scapula   Humerus

↑ The bones of the arm connect into the trunk of the body at the sternum.

Hip joint

If you ask most people where the location of the hip joint is, they will immediately point to the top of the pelvis, usually in the region of the iliac crest. This is not where the joint is at all, but it is often where people bend from. The actual joint is situated much lower in the groin area. When people bend down, however, they will usually try to bend at the top of the iliac crest but in reality they are bending only their back and not the hip joint at all. This action in itself can lead to many problems, including back pain.

The shape of the spine

If you ask people to draw the shape of the spine, many people will draw a gentle S shape. While this is true when standing, the spine actually changes shape when you're sitting or squatting (see image on page 16). Just have a look at a domestic cat – you will see that when it is eating its spine is very straight, yet the spine is very rounded when the cat is lying in front of the fire. At other times, the cat can be seen arching its back. In the same way, our spine changes shape depending on what we are doing. It is sometimes the case that lumbar supports encourage an overarching of the lumbar spine and exacerbate lower back problems.

Location of the lungs

This is another area that many people are confused about. The lungs are in fact very high up in the body and the top of the lung is actually above the collar bone. The lowest part is at the bottom of the rib-cage.

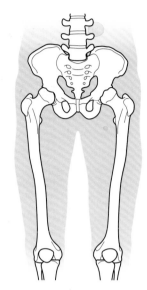

↑ The hip joint is much lower than many people realize.

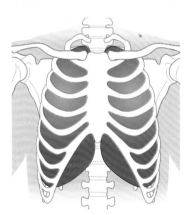

← The lungs extend from above the collar bone to almost the bottom of the rib-cage.

Richard's story

Richard Brennan
Age: 57 | Occupation: Alexander teacher

In my old profession as a driving instructor I spent many hours sitting in a car and, after several years, developed lower back pain. This soon turned into a very painful prolapsed disc, and it was not long before I had shooting pains due to sciatica.

Painkillers and rest brought only temporary relief and became less and less effective. I then saw back specialists who did various tests, but no specific diagnosis could be made. I was told that I would never be able to live a normal life again and I underwent an intensive course of treatment at a residential physiotherapy hospital. Although the staff were doing their best to help, the treatment they gave me only aggravated my condition so my pain was worse than ever.

I started to investigate alternative medicine, including chiropractic, osteopathy, acupuncture, aromatherapy and reiki. While many of these treatments helped to some extent, I could get only short-term relief from the pain.

By chance, I met an Alexander teacher who explained that the Alexander Technique was very effective in helping back sufferers. Although I was very sceptical, I decided to see what it was about. At my first lesson my teacher asked me whether I always sat in the manner that I was currently sitting. He put a mirror in front of me and I could see that I was twisting to the right while leaning to the left at about 20 degrees. This surprised me as I felt perfectly straight. He set about making a few gentle adjustments to the way I was sitting and two things instantly happened: first, I felt completely twisted and, second, my back pain started to abate. He again showed me how I was now sitting in the mirror and I saw that I was now sitting perfectly straight.

I realized that, while teaching people to drive, I had to sit leaning to the left while twisting to the right to see the road ahead and to check if the learner driver was looking in his mirrors and, over the years, this had become my habit wherever I was sitting. As the tensions released during a series of lessons, my back improved, I slept better, my self-esteem and confidence grew and I became happier. Within three months I was leading a normal life again and was lifting and bending without any problem.

I was so impressed and, wanting to help others with similar problems, I trained to be an Alexander teacher myself.

7

Primary Control

Mr Alexander's method lays hold of the individual as a whole, as a self-vitalizing agent. He reconditions and re-educates the reflex mechanisms and brings their habits into normal relation with the functioning of the organism as a whole. I regard this method as thoroughly scientific and educationally sound.

PROFESSOR GEORGE E. COGHILL, ANATOMIST, PHYSIOLOGIST AND
MEMBER OF THE NATIONAL ACADEMY OF SCIENCES U.S.A.

Have you ever stopped for a moment to think about how you actually move around this world? And is it the easiest and most efficient way of going about your activities? Most people do not give the subject any thought whatsoever; in fact it is so alien that at first it is difficult to comprehend what is being asked of us.

We consist of 206 bones, many of which are placed one on top of the other and are irregular in shape. These are suspended by a 'suit' of muscles that supports us and, by maintaining a certain tone, keeps us in an upright position. At the very top of this structure is the head, which weighs 6–7 kg (12–15 lb). This all goes to make our structure extremely unstable, which is great for movement but not so good when we are keeping still.

exercise

FEELING THE WEIGHT

1 Gather together objects that have a combined weight of 7 kg (15 lb); for instance seven bags of sugar or three bags of potatoes.

2 Place them in a container (a box or a bag) and you have the equivalent weight of your own head. It is a very surprising experience when you realize that you are balancing approximately this weight every moment of your waking life.

That is not all. The head is actually set off-balance on top of our spines. Therefore, if we relax the neck muscles, the head is inclined to drop forward. When you watch someone falling asleep while sitting in a chair, the head invariably drops forward and down on to the chest. So, not only are we trying to balance a 7-kg (15-lb) head, but also coping with the fact that its point of balance is not under its centre of gravity (see the illustration, right).

→ **Diagram of the skull and top vertebrae showing the pivot point and the centre of gravity of the head.**

Position of muscles which prevent the head from falling forward

Vertebrae

Skull

Centre of gravity of the head

Pivot point – where the head balances on the spine

exercise

BALANCING A PLATE

1 Take a dinner plate – one you wouldn't mind breaking! Place your finger in the middle of the plate (its centre of gravity), and try to balance the plate using just that one finger.

2 Now repeat the process, but this time place your finger 5 cm (2 in) away from the centre. This is similar to the relationship that the head has to the top of the spine.

At first, this arrangement does not seem to make any sense. Surely if we are to carry around such an incredible weight on top of our spines then it would be sensible for nature to have placed our heads in balance. It is an intriguing puzzle. The answer is simple and yet, at the same time, brilliant.

IMBALANCE OF THE HEAD

The reason that the pivot point of the head is behind its centre of gravity is that, in order to move, all a person has to do is release the muscles at the back of the neck. The head will then go forward slightly and, because of its weight, will take the whole body into movement. In other words, in order to move, a human being has only to let go of the tension in certain muscles and a complex reflex system will do the rest. Most other movements require effort, and the maximum effort is needed at the beginning of the action. For example, a car or aeroplane needs most power when it starts off from a stationary position; it needs relatively little energy to keep it going at a constant speed. Once the head begins to move forward, the body naturally follows.

The implications of this are profound. If we can use ourselves in a more co-ordinated way, our movements will need less effort and thus give us much more energy at the end of the day. This can lead to a more harmonious way of life, as most conflicts and stressful situations are triggered off by fatigue or lack of vitality.

Friends and relatives of Alexander pupils often report a marked change of temperament after only a few lessons. I have heard many comments like, 'John is calmer and much more present these days.'

So the principle of the Alexander Technique is to use our bodies as nature intended; that is, to *decrease* muscular tension in order to move, and not, as most of us do, to increase tension in our muscles. This concept of having to make an effort for movement is reinforced throughout our lives by parents and teachers who tell us: 'You won't get anywhere in this world without making a great deal of effort.' Because of this, we often subconsciously make life much harder than it really needs to be, which is apparent both physically and mentally. By 'letting go' into movement, it is possible to experience how easy and effortless many things can be. Once this starts to permeate our subconscious mind, we are able to be more relaxed in everything we do.

THE INSTABILITY OF THE HUMAN FRAME

As I have said, the skeleton, which consists of over 200 bones mostly assembled one on top of the other, is inherently unstable. It is similar in principle to a pile of children's building blocks – the higher the blocks are placed, the more unstable they become until they actually fall over. This, together with the fact that the head is off-balance, indicates that we have to do very little in order to move. We are designed to 'fall' into movement, and when infants first begin to learn to walk they do just that. They constantly look as though they are about to fall flat on their faces, yet they save themselves just in time by the reflex action of their legs.

Throughout the years, however, because of our unconscious fear of falling, we try to stabilize ourselves by tensing up our muscular system. This, of course, affects our whole physiological system, rendering our reflexes relatively ineffective. As a result, we use excessive muscular effort to perform the action that ought to be done by our reflexes alone.

Each faculty acquires fitness for its function by performing its function; and if its function is performed for it by a substituted agency, none of the required adjustments of nature takes place, but the nature becomes deformed to fit the artificial arrangements instead of the natural arrangements.

HERBERT SPENCER, *THE PRINCIPLES OF ETHICS*

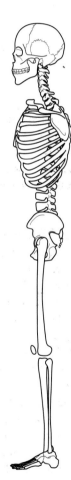

↑ We are, in fact, 206 bones – many of which are placed one on top of the other.

In short, if we do not use ourselves in the way that nature intended, we start to use our muscular mechanisms in a way that will invariably cause unnecessary rigidity of some parts of the body, and an over-relaxation of others. This undue rigidity is always found in those parts of the muscular system that are forced to perform duties other than those intended by nature, and are therefore ill-adapted for their function.

WALKING

When we bear in mind the principles described earlier, walking becomes an action whereby we work *with* gravity rather than against it. Walking is a process of releasing certain muscles that support the head on top of the rest of the body, thus allowing the head to move very slightly forward, but in an upward direction. Since the rest of the body is already in a state of instability, it will then move by slightly falling forward. As soon as the body detects

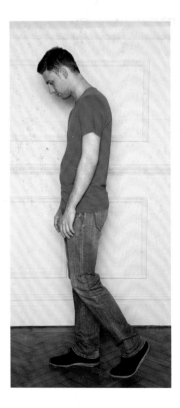 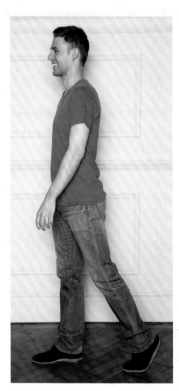

← On the left, the person is looking down, causing tension in his neck and shoulders. On the right, he has his head balanced on top of his spine and is walking with ease.

even the smallest amount of movement, the reflex mechanism automatically and subconsciously bends one knee and sends a leg out in front to save the body from falling over. This is all done completely subconsciously. All you have to do is release muscular tension which is stopping these reflexes from working perfectly. It is important that you do not try to do this.

An important principle emerges when examining the natural way of walking, namely that *the head always leads any movement.*

It is essential to understand this in order to practise the Technique. Every animal, whether it is a snake or an elephant, moves with its head leading – which is why the main sensory organs (eyes, ears, nose and tongue) are all situated in the head. At first, this may seem like an obvious statement, but few human beings apply this principle in movement.

exercise

STEP FORWARD

1 Stand in front of a mirror.

2 Take a step forward.

3 Ask yourself: 'What did I have to do when taking that step?'

4 Notice if you displaced your weight to the left or the right when taking the step. (If you did, it is likely that excess pressure was placed on the hip.)

5 Ask yourself: 'What part of me initiated the movement?'

6 Repeat the exercise several times until you see a pattern emerging.

As you may have discovered, a step is usually taken by lifting the leg with the thigh muscles against the pull of gravity. This, of course, expends unnecessary energy and, if you think about how many steps you take in one day alone, you will realize how much energy is wasted. Not only is there a waste of energy, but also an increase in tension throughout the whole structure simply to

exercise

HOW DO YOU WALK?

1 Slowly allow yourself to fall forward from the ankle joint and save yourself by taking a step.

2 Notice if you have a preference as to which leg you use to save yourself.

3 Are you still inclined to lift the leg rather than let it work by reflex?

4 As you begin to walk, try to notice if you are walking on the outside or the inside of the foot. There should be fairly equal pressure on both sides of each foot. Note any excessive pressure on the inside of the foot, as this can lead to the collapse of the arch.

5 Be aware as you walk of whether your feet have a tendency to point in or out. It is possible that one foot may differ from the other.

6 Be aware of the amount of pressure that is present when your foot comes into contact with the ground.

maintain balance when the foot is raised from the ground. This tension is perfectly harmless if occasional, but when it occurs hundreds of times a day it often leads to rigidity, and eventually this could lead to pain.

I cannot stress too much the importance of not *trying* to change anything; this will always result in an increase of muscular tension and make the situation worse. A change will take place simply by making your habit conscious. This change may not be immediately apparent; you may not notice the difference for a few days or even weeks, so try to be patient. Note: any changes that might come about must be done by applying your direction (see Chapter 5).

THE RIGHT SHOES

People often ask me if I know of a shoe that is good for the feet while walking. The Vivo Barefoot Shoe has been designed with the principles of the Alexander Technique in mind and allows the feet and ankle to work as nature intended (see page 155 for website details). These shoes are not a substitute for learning the Alexander Technique but, with a combination of Alexander lessons and shoes that help the foot to move naturally, you will be able to walk and stand with greater ease.

BENDING DOWN

When bending down to pick up objects, many people do not bend their knees at all; they only bend at the hip joint (that is where the femur connects into the pelvis). This puts an enormous strain on the back muscles, especially those in the lower back area. Without realizing it, most people, when getting up again, are actually picking up half their body weight in addition to the weight of the object. For example, if a person who weighs 67 kg (167 lb) picks up an object which weighs 12.5 kg (28 lb) without bending their knees, they are in fact lifting an extra 44 kg (97 lb) in body weight with their lower back muscles, which will cause considerable tension.

This sort of misuse nearly always leads to lower back pain or, in extreme cases, to a prolapsed disc. If you ever watch professional weightlifters on television, you will see that they always squat when bending, as young children do, using mainly their very powerful thigh and buttock muscles and not the muscles of the back. You will rarely see young children or indigenous people bending down without bending their knees and ankles. Somebody once told me the story about European missionaries in Africa many years ago who were given an African name which, directly translated, meant 'the tribe without knees'.

In the photograph here (see right, below) the woman is perfectly poised and nicely balanced as she lowers herself. Alexander called this a 'position of mechanical advantage'.

POSITION OF MECHANICAL ADVANTAGE

A 'position of mechanical advantage', of which there are a few variations, is the name given by Alexander to describe the body when it is in a state of stability, equilibrium and ease while performing an action that requires a lowering of stature. The word 'position' can be a little confusing as it is not fixed, but a fluid and changeable stance, during which we move our upper body forward as we bend at the hip, knee and ankle joints. We remain in a state of balance while maintaining the length in the spine, avoiding

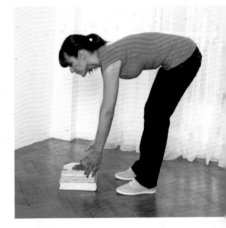

↑ This is how a great many people bend over to pick up things. The whole body is under stress because the top of the body is no longer over its support – the feet.

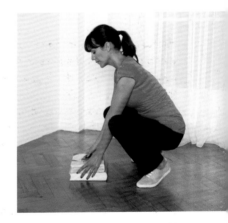

↑ The 'position of mechanical advantage'. As the woman lowers herself she is in balance and is therefore not putting excessive strain on her structure. This position is often seen in children, but hardly ever in adults of developed countries.

arching the lower back or bending the upper spine. As the kinaesthetic sense is often unreliable, it is best to first learn this from a trained Alexander teacher.

Alexander describes the position thus in his first book, *Man's Supreme Inheritance*:

> By my system of obtaining the position of 'mechanical advantage', a perfect system of natural internal massage is rendered possible, such as never before has been attained by orthodox methods, a system which is extraordinarily beneficial in breaking up toxic accumulation; thus avoiding evils which arise from auto-intoxication.

As you become more aware of yourself in different situations, like taking the milk from the fridge or picking up the post in the morning, you will begin to notice a change in the way that you move. Everyday activities become much easier, which of course will be reflected in your attitude to life in general.

exercise

PICK UP A BOOK

1 Place a book on the ground in front of you.

2 Without thinking, pick the book up in your normal way (in other words, in the way which feels most comfortable to you).

3 Repeat several times.

4 Try to notice how you bend down. Do you bend only from the pelvis or do you use your ankle, knee and hip joints simultaneously? If you are bending your knees, how much are you bending them?

5 Try squatting. If you find this hard, just see how far down you can go. Do not force yourself to do more than you can manage. You may need to steady yourself at first by holding on to a nearby chair or table.

It may be useful to re-read Chapter 4 (Inhibition) and Chapter 5 (Directions) and repeat this exercise.

At first this new way of moving may feel strange or even abnormal, because it is outside your habit patterns. However, within a short space of time, the new way becomes natural and the old habits begin to feel unco-ordinated and clumsy.

FROM STANDING TO SITTING

A common habit is to fall backward when sitting down. This excites our fear reflexes unduly and causes us to tense. Also, the legs do not get the exercise they need to keep them in a fit condition. A better way to sit is to go into a bend, as in the photograph below (right), and then gently allow your sitting bones to reach the chair. You should always be able to change your mind and get up at a moment's notice. If you have difficulty with this, simply sit down in the chair as though it might not be there. This can help you to be in balance.

When getting out of a chair we can also put enormous strain on our entire structure, as can be seen in the photographs below (left and middle).

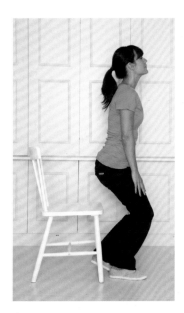

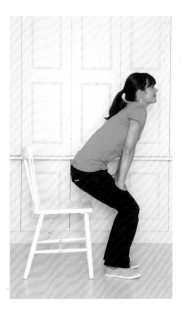

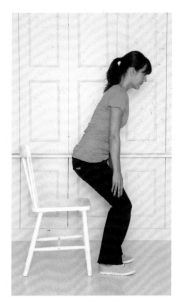

↑ Over-arching the back when sitting will cause you to lose balance and put strain on your spine.

↑ When the body loses balance, it uses muscle tension to save itself.

↑ It is much more beneficial to descend in balance so that the fear reflexes are not triggered.

exercise

SQUATTING

Apart from natural forms of exercise, such as walking, running and swimming, squatting is one of the most useful movements your body can make. As children, all the bending down we do involves squatting, but as we get older we tend to bend our knees less and less. If you are not used to squatting be sure not to overdo it. You can help to balance yourself by holding on to a firm fixture in your home and then gently do some squatting, taking care not to go too far down to begin with.

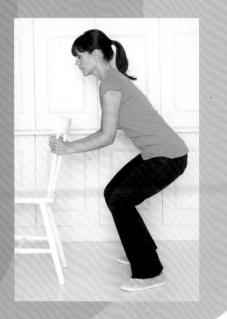

You could also try this when you bend down to pick up objects from the floor. Be sure to take your time as this will help you to observe any excess tension in your body. Be sure that your ankle, knee and hip joints bend simultaneously and that you keep your back straight, although this does not mean that your back is always vertical.

If you have any problems, be sure to consult your Alexander teacher.

MUSCLES AND REFLEXES

Throughout the body we have a complex system of postural reflexes and muscles that support and move us with perfect co-ordination and balance. Most of us, however, misuse these systems and it would be helpful to have an understanding of how these systems work so that we can move through life with greater ease.

We all want good posture, yet many people have differing ideas about the meaning of the word 'posture'. It is often misinterpreted as 'the position in which we hold ourselves while sitting or standing' and that is exactly what people do – they adopt habitual positions and hold these with a huge amount of muscle tension, eventually causing the body to wear out prematurely.

The word 'hold' indicates there is something we have to consciously *do* in order to have good posture, yet a young child has beautiful posture without consciously 'doing' anything to maintain it. It is being maintained by the postural muscles and reflexes, which work below the level of consciousness.

Every adult still has these systems waiting to support, move and keep us in perfect balance as we perform our everyday actions, yet we have got into the habit of using excessive muscle tension, which interferes with these postural reflexes. By learning to release this tension you will be able to move around with much less effort.

MUSCLE

There are more than 650 muscles in the human body and they are responsible for nearly half our body weight. There are basically three kinds of muscle – skeletal, cardiac and smooth. The Alexander Technique is directly concerned with the first type – skeletal – but this may well have an indirect effect on the other two muscle types. Although the bones form the framework for the body, they cannot move by themselves.

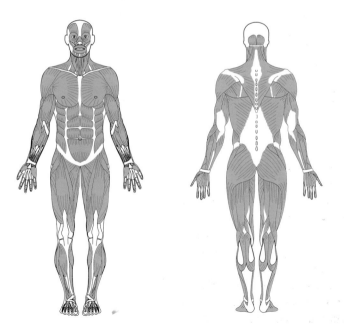

← We have a 'suit' of muscles that support and move us in all our actions.

Muscles vary greatly in size, from the huge gluteus (buttock muscles) to the minute stapedius muscles found in the ear. Skeletal muscle is the tissue that joins two or more bones together and because of its power of contraction and relaxation, a movement can be initiated or a position maintained. Skeletal muscles may have two or more points of attachment. For example, the biceps join the shoulder blade (scapula) to the lower arm (radius), or they may join three bones together – as in the case of the sterno-cleido mastoid muscle, which joins the head (the mastoid process of the temporal bone) to the clavicle and the front of the rib-cage (sternum).

MUSCLE CONTRACTION

It is important to note that muscles can only pull two bones toward each other, but can never push them apart – the only way muscles can move bones away from one another is simply to stop contracting. This is why muscles work in pairs: one is the mover (the one in a state of contraction) and is known as the agonist muscle, while the other (which slowly relaxes to allow controlled movement) is called the antagonistic muscle. Every muscle takes its turn at being the agonist and then the antagonist. Muscles are in fact co-operating with each other all the time in a *slight* state of

⬇ **Diagrams of the forearm moving downward (left) and upward (right), showing agonist and antagonistic action.**

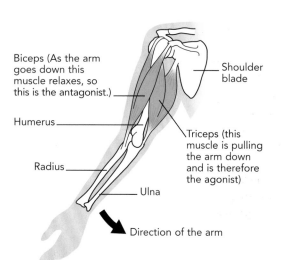

Biceps (As the arm goes down this muscle relaxes, so this is the antagonist.)

Humerus

Radius

Shoulder blade

Triceps (this muscle is pulling the arm down and is therefore the agonist)

Ulna

Direction of the arm

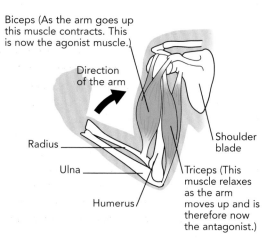

Biceps (As the arm goes up this muscle contracts. This is now the agonist muscle.)

Direction of the arm

Radius

Ulna

Humerus

Shoulder blade

Triceps (This muscle relaxes as the arm moves up and is therefore now the antagonist.)

tension, which is what gives them their tone. The only part of the muscle that does not contract is the connection between bone and the contractile tissue, commonly known as the tendon.

TYPES OF MUSCLE FIBRES

Different muscles perform different functions and, as a consequence, differ in structure and colour. All muscle has a variety of different muscle fibres but, if a muscle has a specific function, it will have a majority of a certain type of fibres. For the purpose of simply understanding the differences, we can split the muscles into two groups, known anatomically as fast twitch and slow twitch according to the speed at which they contract.

Fast twitch

These muscle fibres contract quickly and are used in rapid movements such as walking, running and picking things up. The majority of these muscles are found in the 'activity muscles' such as the arms and legs.

Slow twitch

These muscle fibres contract relatively slowly, but are resistant to fatigue and can work for long periods without rest. They are found predominantly in the deep postural muscles of the trunk and legs.

Therefore, one of the most significant differences between the different types of muscle fibres is that the ones we use to maintain posture are much more fatigue – resistant than the ones we use for movement. As most people try to improve their posture by conscious thought – such as pulling their shoulders back or sitting up straight – they are in fact using their fast twitch muscles, which get tired after a few minutes. So even with all good intentions, it is physically impossible to improve good posture by merely tensing our muscles. We can, however, improve our posture and the way we 'use ourselves' generally by releasing muscular tension and letting the postural reflexes work. This is what Alexander was referring to when he said that if you stop doing the wrong thing, the right thing will happen by itself.

HOW MUSCLES CONTRACT

As you can see in the illustration below, muscles are composed of bundles (fascicles) of muscle cells (or fibres), each enclosed in a partition of fibrous tissue known as the perimysium. These partitions are again surrounded by an outer sheath of tissue known as the fascia (or epimysium). When carefully examined, these bundles of muscle cells, which can be up to 20 cm (8 in) in length, are found to consist of a further collection of fibres which form the units of muscle. It is at this cellular level that the results of practising the Alexander Technique can be discerned.

These fibres (or myofibrils), shorten when chemically activated, which occurs in response to nervous stimuli. The chemical that initiates this depends on the type of muscle, but the response is always the same – namely a shortening of protein molecules.

If muscles are in a constant state of tension, the body will adapt, leading to a shortening of the whole muscle, as can be illustrated by women who frequently wear high heels. Due to a continual state of contraction of the calf muscle, the muscle becomes shorter and in some cases women can find it difficult to reach the ground with their heels when they are not wearing high-heeled shoes.

Even thinking of lengthening and widening can bring about an increase in length of the muscle fibres, and if this is continued over a period of time it can result in an overall lengthening of the body. As I have mentioned before, there are many reports of people who have increased in height by 2.5 cm (1 in) or more during the course of Alexander lessons. But do not worry, this process happens over weeks or months – it is very gradual and gentle!

It is important to note that any excess muscular tension is bound to pull bones out of place (such as a shoulder blade that protrudes rather than rests comfortably on the rib-cage), which will in turn cause other muscles to be unnecessarily taut. As a result, one tense muscle is bound to affect the whole organism.

A prolonged increase in muscle tension can also result in interference in the nervous, digestive, respiratory and circulatory systems, and will inevitably impair natural functions.

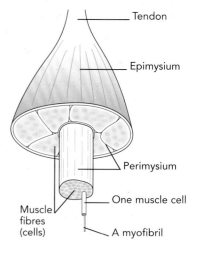

↑ **The structure of a skeletal muscle.**

THE CIRCULATORY OR VASCULAR SYSTEM

This system consists of arteries, veins and capillaries through which an equivalent of 36,000 litres (8,000 gallons) of blood is pumped every single day. The total length of the blood vessels is an amazing 102,500 km or 64,000 miles which, if stretched out, would go around the Earth twice over!

The arteries and veins, like the nerves, weave in and out between the muscles of the body. They are not rigid tubes, but are able to contract and dilate to let a larger or smaller amount of blood flow through at just the right pressure. If the muscles through which the blood vessels pass are particularly taut, this obviously restricts the flow of the blood and the heart will then have to work harder to compensate, or parts of the body will be deprived of the nourishment that the blood supplies. This pressure on the arteries and veins could be a major contributing factor in various health problems.

THE RESPIRATORY SYSTEM

One of the most noticeable things about my students is they have almost all had a habit of shallow breathing. In fact many people take in only about a quarter of the air that a 'normal' breath should supply. The average adult breathes roughly 13,650 litres (2,800 gallons) of air each day, so it is essential that this system works effectively and efficiently. The reason people suffer from shallow breathing is that they:

- Sit in a slumped fashion, which constricts their lung capacity.
- Sit in a rigid fashion, so their rib-cage is relatively fixed.
- Over-tighten their intercostal muscles (the muscles which connect one rib to another).
- Shorten their back muscles which in turn causes the rib movement to be restricted.
- Over-tense the back muscles which in turn will shorten the spine. This will cause a compression on the joint which connects the ribs to the vertebrae and results in a restriction of movement of the whole rib-cage.

From the exercise on page 92 it is easy to see that excess muscular activity (or lack of it) will directly affect breathing patterns.

exercise

BREATHING PATTERNS

1 Sit in a chair and just notice your breathing: where are you breathing from? Is your breathing shallow or deep? Which part of your body has the most movement?

2 Now sit in a slumped fashion – the more slumped the better!

3 Take a deep breath and note how much air you are able to take in.

4 This time sit in a very rigid and upright position, as 'straight' as you possibly can.

5 Again, take a very deep breath and be aware of how much air is taken in.

6 Lastly, sit in a way that is neither slumped nor rigid and take a breath.

7 Compare the three results, which should speak for themselves.

THE DIGESTIVE SYSTEM

The whole digestive system relies heavily on the muscles of the body to perform its natural functions – whether it is the jaw muscles which aid the teeth in chewing food or the muscular contractions (peristalsis) that force the food along the digestive tract. In fact, the whole of the stomach is a large muscular sac. Since, as I have said before, tension in one muscle will invariably affect the whole muscular system, the efficient functioning of the processes of digestion, absorption and assimilation will depend on the overall freedom of the entire muscular system.

THE SKELETAL SYSTEM

Any muscular tension can affect the movement of the entire body, which can cause a restriction of the synovial joints, the most common and most movable joints in the body. The dynamics of joint nutrition rely on the movements of the joint to cause the pressure within the joint to drop. This, in turn, causes blood plasma to be released into the joint, which is essential for more synovial fluid to be formed. The process is essential for efficient lubrication of the joint. A good example of this can be seen in people in India who rarely lose their ability to squat, even in old age, because they have not lost the movement in their joints – and the more movement in the joints, the more synovial fluid is produced.

Bone is a very hard substance indeed, which can last for many centuries, so you can imagine the amount of force that the muscles exert when two bones are pulled together and start to wear each other down, as in the case of arthritis.

Because every single bone of the skeleton is interconnected by the muscles, if we habitually have excess tension within our structure we are, in reality, pulling one part of ourselves down onto another part. This, of course, is detrimental to our balance, co-ordination and poise and, eventually, to our total wellbeing, both physical and mental.

THE NERVOUS SYSTEM

The nervous, or neurological, system consists of a network of nerve fibres which run from the brain and the spinal cord (together referred to as the central nervous system) to the rest of the body. The function of this system is to convey messages to and from every part of the organism.

Many of the nerve fibres pass between muscle and bone, as well as between one muscle and another. If, due to stress, a muscle

exercise

MUSCLE TENSION

To demonstrate how hard a muscle may become under tension:

1 Feel your biceps (the muscles of the upper arm) as your arm hangs freely.

2 Pick up a heavy weight, such as a chair, with only one arm.

3 Note the difference.

is in a permanent state of contraction, a nerve can become trapped by the hardened muscle and produce a great deal of pain, such as sciatica. The pain will, of course, cause the person to tense up even more, thus creating a vicious cycle. Anyone who has experienced a trapped nerve of any description will tell you how painful it is.

REFLEXES

A reflex action, or reflex, is an involuntary and nearly instantaneous movement in response to a stimulus. When there is a change in length or loading of a muscle, specialized nerve endings called mechanoreceptors are stimulated. There are three categories of reflexes:

Superficial reflexes

These comprise any sudden movements which result when the skin is lightly brushed or pricked. Example: The bending movement of the toes when the sole of the foot is stroked firmly from heel to sole.

Deep reflexes

These are dependent upon the constant state of mild contraction which the muscles are in when at rest. Example: The patella reflex, more commonly known as the knee-jerk, which occurs when the tendon of the muscle is tapped sharply.

Visceral reflexes

These are reflexes that are connected with the various organs of the body. Example: The narrowing of the pupil when a bright light is shone directly into the eye.

All reflex actions occur without any conscious control, yet in some cases they can be overridden by reasoning. If you pick up a hot plate, the reflex action is to drop the plate on to the floor, but our reasoning intelligence knows this will result in a mess on the floor, so the plate is placed down on the table nearby. (This will, of course, depend on how hot the plate is!) It seems that, in animals, reflex actions are much more powerful than reasoning. For example, if a cat is chased by a dog it may well run across a busy road in an attempt to escape, which can lead to tragic consequences. A human being, on the other hand, when being chased will sum up the advantages and disadvantages of running out into the road. In this way, our rational intelligence can indeed prove sounder than the reflex.

We have reflexes because there are thousands of adjustments that have to be made each minute and we cannot possibly think of them all with our conscious brain. We can, however, still carry out various activities (such as carrying, bending, walking or reaching out) that, by rights, should upset our balance and cause us to topple over, if it were not for our muscular system making continuous adjustments of tension and position through our reflexes.

Overleaf are four examples of how the use or misuse of ourselves can affect some of the major reflexes.

STRETCH REFLEXES IN CONNECTION WITH THE ALEXANDER TECHNIQUE

A stretch reflex is an instantaneous contraction when the muscles are stretched too far or too quickly. The stretch may be caused by a stimulus, such as the upward pressure of the intervertebral discs of the spine, or by an external force such as gravity. The function of the stretch reflex is to stop one part of the body dislocating from the rest of the structure if it is suddenly or unexpectedly pulled – a similar action to the inertia-reel seat belts used in most cars today.

In other words, if a muscle is pulled too suddenly or too far, the effect will be to shorten still further. This begs the question whether traction can in some cases cause a shortening of the structure.

In *Body Awareness in Action*, Professor Frank Pierce Jones writes:

> The tendency of the body to lengthen from within gives it strength as well as buoyancy. If the discs have expanded, the small muscles attached to the vertebrae must have been lengthened and their strength thereby increased. The lengthening and strengthening initiated by the discs and the small muscles would be transmitted by purely mechanical means to the longer muscles, and the process would continue to the surface. This lengthening-strengthening process is further enhanced by movement. In moving the body or one of its parts against gravity, the lifting muscles are facilitated by the stretch placed upon them by the part that is being lifted (a movement against gravity is facilitated by gravity itself). In getting up from a chair, for example, the head, neck and back move forward as a unit without losing their length. In the process, the muscles in the lower back, buttocks and thighs are stretched. When the stretch reaches

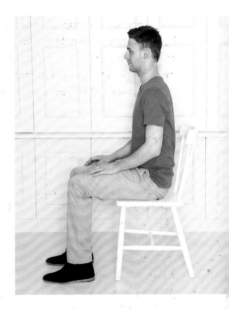

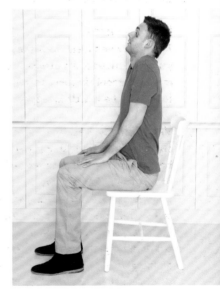

⬆ The person at the top is sitting in a relaxed way. When the fear reflex is triggered, the shoulders hunch, the head is retracted backward and the back becomes arched (bottom).

exercise

TESTING THE FEAR REFLEX

1 Place your hands so that they rest on the back of the neck with the middle fingers just touching.

2 Stand with your back to a sofa as though you were about to sit down.

3 Now sit down by falling backward, while trying to notice any pressure on your hands.

exercise

TESTING THE TOE REFLEXES

You can test these reflexes very easily for yourself:

1 Ask a friend to sit in a chair.

2 Make sure they are sitting erect. Place a hand on their knee and move their leg from side to side. It should move quite easily.

3 Now ask them to lean forward so more of their weight is on their feet and less on their sitting bones.

4 Again place your hand on their knee, and try to move their leg from side to side once again. This time the leg should not move so easily.

Because more weight is on the toes, the nerve endings between the toes are activated, causing the leg muscles to tighten, ready for the standing position.

a certain level of intensity, the stretched muscles contract reflexly, straightening the hip joint and in turn stretching the muscles around the knee. The body is thus lifted smoothly and easily with a sense of little or no effort.

This is the sort of experience a pupil has during an Alexander lesson, referred to as 'the Alexander experience'.

exercise

MOVING WITH LESS EFFORT

1 Sit on a kitchen chair.

2 Stand up in your normal way.

3 Sit down again, in your usual manner.

4 Now stand up again, but this time move your torso in one piece from the hip joints, with a sense of slightly falling forward out of the chair.

5 As you sit down, again think about bending forward from the hips with a sense of falling forward. Make sure you also bend your knees.

6 Repeat this process a few times and you will begin to see how you can move with less effort. You may feel a greater sense of balance by doing it in a new way, but be aware that you may have Faulty Sensory Awareness, so it is a good idea to use a mirror.

exercise

USING THE RIGHT MUSCLES?

Most people try to improve their posture with their fast twitch muscles instead of their postural muscles. Since the fast twitch muscles are designed for activity, they will tire easily, making permanent change impossible, as you will see from this exercise.

1 Stand or sit in front of a mirror as before.

2 See if you can notice anything about your posture that you would like to change.

3 If you can, put yourself into a position that you are happy with.

4 Wait for a few minutes so that you can see whether your muscles begin to tire. If they do, you know that you have increased muscular tension to improve your posture instead of releasing it.

The different reflexes

THE FALLING REFLEX

Whenever our structure is off-balance and we are likely to fall backward, the fear reflex, sometimes known as the 'startle pattern' is activated. This is not unlike the reflex action which is brought about by a sudden loud noise. It is interesting to observe that this reaction is most noticeable in the neck muscles and nowhere else. The head is pulled backward as the muscles shorten and the shoulders become hunched, the very actions recognized by Alexander as being habits common to all humans. There is good reason for this response to falling backward; it protects the lower parts of the brain, the cerebellum and the medulla, as well as the top of the spinal cord. Any damage to these areas would render a person incapacitated for life. Most of us, however, trigger this reflex every time we sit down in a chair because, when sitting down, we tend to fall back for at least part of the way.

It is likely that you felt your neck muscles stiffen when you tried the above exercise – this is the fear reflex which is often unnecessarily activated every time we sit or stand, until it becomes a constant habit.

THE PATELLA REFLEX

This is perhaps the most well-known reflex in the body. Doctors use it to test a reflex system by tapping gently on the tendon just below the patella (kneecap). Striking the patellar tendon just below the patella stretches the quadriceps muscles in the thigh and this stimulates stretch sensory receptors, causing an impulse in a sensory nerve fibre of the femoral nerve leading to the lumbar region of the spinal cord. There, the sensory neuron synapses directly with a motor neuron that causes a contraction of the quadriceps femoris muscle. This contraction, co-ordinated with the relaxation of the antagonistic flexor hamstring muscle, causes the leg to kick. This reflex helps maintain posture and balance, allowing one to walk without consciously thinking about each step.

THE POSTURAL REFLEXES OF THE FEET

Dr David Garlick, a senior lecturer in physiology at the University of New South Wales in Sydney, has shown that many of the involuntary muscles in the torso are activated by sensory nerve endings in the feet. These nerve endings are sensitive to pressure, so the more weight there is on our feet the better these muscles and reflexes will work. (This happens even when sitting down if the soles of the feet are on the ground – though obviously not to the same extent.) However, as I have said before, many people do not position their feet in a balanced way when they stand; they tend to put too much weight on either their heels or their toes or, alternatively, put most of their weight on one side.

In such cases, the sensory nerve endings cannot be stimulated, and there will be much less input of the postural muscles which automatically keep us erect. As a result, we start to use our fast twitch muscles instead and, because they tire very quickly, it will be an effort for us to maintain an upright posture; after a while we inevitably begin to slump.

Re-education, using the principles of the Technique, can start to restore the body's rightful balance, thus encouraging the appropriate muscles to be used for the appropriate purpose.

THE TOE REFLEXES

Between the metatarsal bones of the foot, which end as the five toes, there are four sets of muscles called the dorsal interossei. Attached to each of these muscles there are sensory nerve endings, which activate the muscles of the leg. Like the postural reflexes, these operate mainly when standing. If, as before, we are not standing evenly on our feet, these reflexes will not work effectively and once again we will have to involve our voluntary system, which requires much more effort.

8

Goal Orientation

*Pleasure in the job puts
perfection in the work.*

ARISTOTLE

END-GAINING

What Alexander called 'end-gaining', we today call 'goal orientation'. This is the fundamental approach of our educational system, and the habits we learn at school permeate the rest of our life.

> Give a child conscious control and you give him poise, the essential starting point for education. Without that poise, which is a result aimed at by neither the old nor the new methods of education, he will presently be cramped and distorted by his environment.
> **FREDERICK MATTHIAS ALEXANDER**

The 'end-gaining' approach seems to permeate every sphere of life. As a species, we try to make our lives more comfortable and enjoyable. This is only natural. Yet it is just as natural to look at the consequences of the actions as we bring about a desired end. In other words, we need to pay attention to the way in which we achieve any particular goal. Alexander called this considering 'the means whereby'. When we fail to do so we are often heading for trouble.

Just consider for a moment the pollution that we create every single day. I remember a TV programme in 1968 called 'Owing To Lack of Interest Tomorrow Has Been Cancelled'. Since then, we have had so much information about global warming and the effects that pollution is having on our planet, yet we go on making the same mistakes over and over again, even though the results of our actions are pointed out so clearly. The greenhouse effect, which is threatening every species on the planet, including ourselves, is a perfect example of global 'end-gaining'.

Alexander wrote in his last book:

> Man knows all about the means whereby he can keep the in-animate machine in order, and considers it his duty to make proper use of these, but he knows little or nothing about the means whereby he can keep in order that animate human machine – himself. The great majority of people have not yet awakened to the great and growing need of such a 'means whereby' and so have not yet appreciated that these are essential to the art of living healthily, happily and in harmony with one another.

Is it not strange that man has become so skilled in the nature and workings of the machines he has created and yet knows so little about the mechanisms of his own organism?

THE MEANS WHEREBY

It is necessary for us to have goals in life and to attain them; this is only human. It is what we do in the process that we need to look at. The way we go about our everyday activities is a reflection of what we do to our planet. After all, if we do not respect ourselves, how are we ever going to respect the planet on which we live? Attending to the means whereby any end is attained is a case of stopping for a moment and thinking things through to their natural conclusion.

Trying to gain an end without thinking of the best way for that end to be attained can become a habit – a habit of living for the future rather than being in the present moment. Achieving a goal by considering each step of the way in a conscious manner encourages us to remain in the present and, as a result, we are far more likely to achieve the end that we set out to accomplish. Attending to the 'means whereby' does not mean being over careful, slow or cautious; it means applying common sense to the situation.

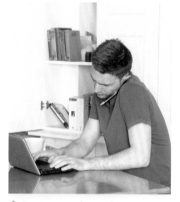

↑ During our busy day, we often become completely unaware of ourselves.

TRYING TOO HARD

When you think carefully about the way in which actions are performed, the old saying, 'When at first you don't succeed, try, try, and try again' becomes, 'When at first you don't succeed, never try again… at least not in the same way.'

Trying invariably involves excessive and unnecessary tension. It was only when Alexander gave up trying so hard that he was able to achieve the end he had been trying to reach for many years, namely to stop pulling his head back when he talked.

When I give this exercise at my classes, it is surprising how many people cannot think of more than three or four ways of achieving their goal. If you have the same problem, here are a few different ways you can use: running, walking, crawling, hopping, skipping, tip-toeing, stomping and jumping,

If you take walking, for instance, there are so many different ways in which you can walk: fast, medium, slow (with many variations in between), in a straight line, in an arc, in a zig-zag, forward, backward, sideways, while leaning sideways, while leaning backward, while leaning forward, while twisting from side to side.

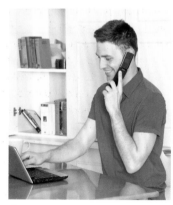

↑ Whatever job we may do, it is important to consider the way we use ourselves.

You can, of course, combine one or more of the above; for example you could tip-toe slowly sideways, but in a straight line, while you are slightly leaning forward! There is a vast number of combinations possible.

exercise

UNDERSTANDING END-GAINING

This simple procedure will help you to understand what is meant by end-gaining and by being more conscious while in activity.

1 Find yourself a spacious area such as a large room or, better still, a garden.

2 Go to one end of the room or garden and choose an object at the other. Then, without thinking, go and touch that object.

3 Repeat the same procedure, only this time before you go to the object, decide how you are going to reach that object.

4 Repeat this process several times, choosing a different way each time.

The first way would be your habitual way, with no conscious means applied, but the other ways, of which there are thousands of variations, were performed by a conscious 'means whereby'.

Another exercise is to think of a completely different way of moving that is not mentioned above. If you want to watch someone who is expert at varying their movements, just watch a young child and you will be amazed how often they change their style of moving. One moment they are walking, the next they are skipping, then they run for a few steps, and so on.

Take the example of walking once again: see how many different ways you can think of to get from 'A' to 'B'. Enjoy finding the many thousands of possible ways that your body has of moving. At first you may quickly run out of ideas but, when you become more experienced, there is a wide range of ways in which you can move.

The problem for us all is that, in order to be more conscious, we have to start living in a new way. The principles of inhibition and direction must be applied instead of the hazardous end-gaining behaviour that has become habitual. Like everything else, you cannot rush the process and we must be content with a steady progress. It is easy to become anxious about being on the right track, even though what we perceive as right is often wrong. However, with patience, you will continue to improve as you learn to consciously attend to the means whereby you perform your day-to-day activities.

9

The Force of Habit

_We can throw away the habit of a lifetime
in a few minutes if we use our brains._

FREDERICK MATTHIAS ALEXANDER

At any given moment in our waking life our senses take in information from the outside world to our brain, so that we can make conscious choices. Yet, how truly conscious are we about what goes on around us most of the time? We tend to be thinking about what has happened in the past or what may happen in the future. Many of us are rarely living in the present. This is because from an early age we are actively encouraged to think about the future.

While we are thinking of the past or the future we cannot attend to the present – to think about the activity we are performing. We cannot make conscious choices and we therefore have to revert to a habitual and automatic mode of behaviour. In order to practise the Alexander Technique effectively we have to be present and in the here and now. This enables us to make conscious choices in our daily lives which results in the heightening of our awareness so our senses become more acute.

If the exercise overleaf is performed properly you should see, hear, smell, touch and taste things around you more acutely. We tend to miss a great deal of our lives because we have cultivated this habit of paying too little attention to what we are doing in the present moment. This is to our detriment physically, mentally, emotionally and spiritually.

Have you ever been on your way to a shop and walked straight past because you were busy thinking about something else? Or driven past the turning to the road you live on and not realized until minutes later? I am sure you have, as it a common experience. Alexander called this 'the mind-wandering habit'.

An old friend and teacher once said, 'The Creator gives man the gift of thought. But what man thinks about is his own gift to himself.' We always have the choice of what to think about, but we usually let our thoughts run wild and, when we do try to exercise some control, we find it almost impossible. Really being present and not mind-wandering does take practise, but I assure you that perseverance will reap great rewards.

HABITS

The dictionary definition of the word 'habit' is 'the behaviour that is guided by an automatic reaction to a specific situation'.

There are two types of habit to be considered – conscious and unconscious. Some of these habits are completely harmless, others may be beneficial but, on the whole, habits tend to be detrimental

exercise

PAYING ATTENTION TO THE PRESENT

1 Take a walk in the countryside or in a nearby park.

2 Be aware of your sense of sight. For about five minutes, look around and see what you can see… the trees, the clouds, the grass, and so on.

3 Write down your experience.

4 Then be aware of your sense of hearing… what can you hear? Maybe the wind in the trees, perhaps a child laughing or crying, or the birds singing.

5 Again, write down your experiences.

6 Now turn your attention to your sense of smell… what can you smell?

7 And now to feeling… feel the wind in your hair, the air on your face, or even the breath going in and out of your lungs and your heart beating in your chest.

8 Lastly, pay attention to the kinaesthetic senses. These 'inside' senses tell you where you are in space. Without reacting to the information that you are sensing, ask yourself how you feel when you are moving. Do you sense that you are straight, leaning forward or backward? Do you feel that you are leaning to the left or right? Although you cannot really know for certain if what you are feeling is correct without a mirror, it is useful to become more aware of this sense.

9 When you get home, go to the kitchen and make yourself something to eat and focus all your attention on your sense of taste… the texture of the food, the flavours, and so on.

10 Take some time to see if you were more aware than you usually are.

to a person's natural and spontaneous way of being. By being aware of your habits, you are able to alter them if you choose.

We will all have some, if not all, of the above habits and, in order to bring about a desirable change in ourselves, we must make the unconscious conscious. It is impossible to change a habit while it is still below our level of consciousness. It is vital to recognize the implications of long-term habits of use on our health and happiness.

Conscious and unconscious habits

CONSCIOUS HABITS

These are habits that we are already aware of, such as:

- Always sitting in the same chair.
- Always having meals at the same time each day.
- Smoking.
- Drinking.
- Cleaning your teeth after every meal.
- Biting your fingernails.
- Fidgeting.
- Leaving the top off the toothpaste.

UNCONSCIOUS HABITS

These are the habits of use to which Alexander constantly referred. They include:

- Stiffening the neck muscles.
- Bracing the knees back.
- Arching the back in an excessive manner.
- Gripping the floor with the toes.
- Pushing the hips forward.
- Tensing up the shoulders.
- Pulling back the head.
- Holding the rib-cage rigid.

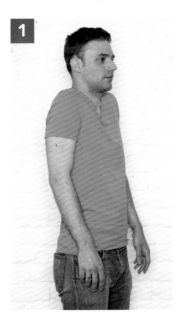

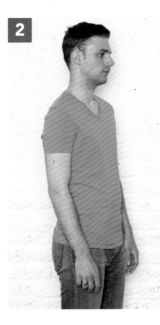

← 1. It is hard to believe, but many people tend to hunch their shoulders, yet are completely unaware of it. 2. With a little awareness, we can easily let go of this habit.

In his book *Body Awareness in Action*, Professor Frank Pierce Jones writes:

> Habits are not 'an untied bundle' of isolated acts. They interact with one another and together make up an integrated whole.

Whether or not a particular habit is manifest, it is always operative and contributes to character and personality. A man may give himself away in a look or a gesture. A habit cannot be changed without intelligent control of an appropriate means or mechanism. To believe that it can is to believe in magic. People still think, nevertheless, that by passing laws, or by 'wishing hard enough' or 'feeling strongly enough' they can change human behaviour and get a desirable result. That is superstition.

He then goes on to quote the philosopher John Dewey:

> The real opposition is not between reason and habit, but between routine or unintelligent habit and intelligent habit or art. Old habits need modification no matter how good they have been. It is the function of intelligence to determine where changes should be made.

How are you sitting?

Habits often arise when we are unconscious of the things around us. Try to be aware of how you are sitting. See if you can notice whether you continually repeat the same positions over and over again. Ask yourself the following questions:

- Do you have your left leg crossed over the right leg, or do you tend to cross your right leg over the left?
- What position are your feet in?
- What are you doing with your arms and hands?
- Do you have your arms folded or your hands clenched together?
- Are you sitting with your head on one side?

Even asking yourself these questions can help you to become more aware of certain habits. To become more aware of your own personal habits try the exercise opposite:

exercises

WHAT'S YOUR HABIT?

1 Stand up with your weight evenly distributed on both feet.

2 Now shift the weight on to your right leg so that you are sinking down into your right hip, making sure your left foot is still on the ground.

3 Now reverse the procedure by sinking down into your left hip.

4 Whichever of these two feels more comfortable is your habit.

ARMS FOLDED

1 Ask a friend to fold his arms; he will probably do this without thinking.

2 Notice which arm is in front of the other.

3 Ask him to fold his arms in the opposite fashion (i.e. the front arm now becomes the back arm).

4 Nine people out of 10 find this quite difficult; check your friend has in fact folded his arms in the opposite way.

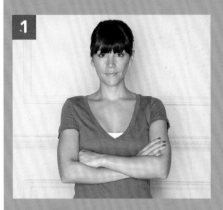 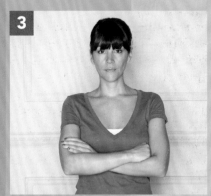

LEMON SQUEEZING

Try squeezing a lemon or an orange with the hand you use the least (usually the left hand as most people are right-handed).

THE POWER OF HABIT

Here is an interesting and true story about the power of habit, which happened in the US some years ago.

A policeman was waiting near a traffic light at 4 am when a car drove through the lights the other way. The policeman looked up, saw a red light and thought the car had jumped the lights, which of course it had not. He sped after the car with his siren sounding and pulled it over. The driver asked, 'What have I done wrong?' The officer, realizing that he had made a mistake, replied, 'You went through a green light.' Because the driver had a strong habit of being defensive with figures of authority, he responded by saying, 'No, I didn't. No, I didn't. I am absolutely sure it was red!'

Our physical habits invariably stem from the rigid way we think, which is often due to preconceived ideas and baseless assumptions. When we change the patterns of movement, we are also altering the way we think. By understanding and applying those principles we are able to eradicate our numerous harmful habits.

CHOICES

There is an old saying, 'When things go wrong, don't go with them.' But we have to make a conscious choice about what we are going to do at any given moment in time. The freedom to make a real choice leads to the freedom of the spirit which is inherent in every one of us. This freedom is essential to regain dignity and integrity which would lead man to reclaiming his rightful place as 'The Crown of Creation'.

One of Alexander's main teachings was that, even after making an initial choice, we should remain open to 're-choose' at any time.

Choice is: the power to make a decision based on reason and discrimination rather than out of fear or habit.

I remember seeing a picture of a queue of lemmings waiting to jump off a cliff with the caption, '2,000 lemmings can't be wrong!' Once, as I was driving home in heavy traffic, I turned left and the car behind me must have thought I knew a short cut. Other drivers evidently presumed the same and eventually eight cars followed me. You can imagine their surprise when I parked my car at the end of a cul-de-sac! An amusing event, but many people follow others instead of thinking for themselves. In a survey in post-war Germany, people were asked, 'Why did you personally go to war?' Nearly all of them said, 'Because everyone else was going – I didn't want to go at all.'

This next exercise may seem like a long-winded way of going

exercise

THE SECRET OF FREE CHOICE

This exercise demonstrates the Alexander Technique in a nutshell, but is most beneficial if done after a few lessons.

1 Choose an action, any one will do, but for the sake of the exercise try raising your arm out in front of you until it is level with your shoulder.

2 Inhibit any immediate response to raise your arm.

3 Give yourself the following instruction: think of your neck being free so that your head is going forward and upward lengthening and widening your back.

4 Continue to project this direction until you believe that you are sufficiently conversant with it to achieve the aim of lifting your arm without tightening your neck muscles.

5 While continuing to think of your direction, stop and consciously reconsider your initial decision. Ask yourself whether you will after all go on to perform the action of lifting your arm, or will you not? Or will you do something else altogether such as lifting your leg, for example.

6 Then and there make a fresh decision. Either:

   a Not to go ahead and gain your original 'end', in which case continue to give yourself the directions laid down in Step 3.

   b To decide to do something different altogether (say, lifting the leg instead of lifting the arm), in which case continue to give your direction while you carry out this last decision and actually lift the leg.

   c To go ahead and lift the arm, in which case continue to project your direction to maintain your new 'use' and then perform the action of lifting the arm.

about a simple action, but here lies the secret of *free choice*. With practise it can be accomplished very swiftly.

In all three choices that you make the essence was to:

Stop
Make a decision
But at all times continue to give yourself the directions.

Remember: If you do what you have always done… you will get what you have always got.

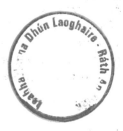

10

Body, Mind and Emotional Unity

You translate everything, whether physical or mental or spiritual, into muscular tension.

FREDERICK MATTHIAS ALEXANDER

Many of the early philosophers realized that the mind, body and emotions were all interconnected. Hippocrates, 'the father of modern medicine', came to the conclusion 2,500 years ago that a human being's health is directly related to his natural surroundings; he was a firm believer that the healing of the body cannot be separated from the health of mind and emotions. He stated that, with the right mental and emotional conditions, the body had a natural ability to heal itself. In a similar way, Plato was convinced that 'the cure of the parts should not be attempted without the treatment of the whole', while Socrates declared: 'To do is to be.'

In Alexander's time, however, much of this ancient wisdom had almost been forgotten. The mind, the body and the emotions were often treated as very separate entities. Mental hospitals were very different from hospitals dealing with physical ailments and, to a large extent, they still are today. Even with all our amazing advances in medicine it is often still the case that the physical area of pain is treated without much consideration of the body as a whole, let alone by taking into account the mental or emotional condition of the patient as well. So, Alexander was required to rediscover some fundamental and ancient laws.

REDISCOVERING FUNDAMENTAL LAWS

During the observations of himself, Alexander realized that every part of his body was interconnected with every other part. He noticed that, when he stopped pulling his head back, his toes relaxed onto the ground – he had experienced it without doubt. This showed him that everything between his head and his feet was being affected, yet many therapies today still ignore this fundamental principle.

If someone has a problem with their back it is their back alone that is examined and treated, yet pain is often referred to different parts of the body. In my experience as an Alexander teacher, many back, hip, knee or ankle problems are directly caused by the pulling back of the head onto the spine or someone may have a neck or shoulder problem because of the way they are standing on their feet.

The next realization Alexander had was that, when he was able to release the tension in his neck that was at the root of his voice problem, the breathing problems that had affected his health all his life disappeared. Through his experience with both himself

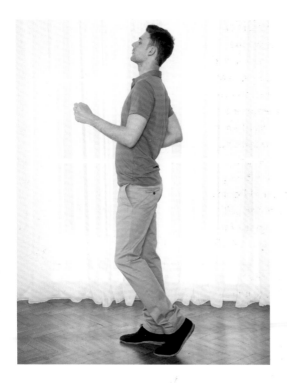

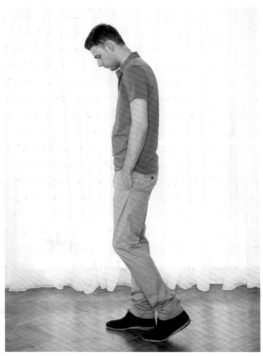

↑ **Different states of mind can produce very different ways of moving.**

and others, Alexander became convinced that the body, mind and emotions not only affected one another, they were in fact inseparable. They were merely different facets of the same entity.

This simple, fundamental principle means that, if we change one thing, we change all of them. It is easy to see this principle all around us. For example, the posture of a footballer who is walking off the pitch after losing a match is totally different to the way that same footballer moves when he has just won the match. The way people stand at a bus stop waiting to go to work is very different from the way those people stand in a queue at the airport when they are going on holiday. When I used to teach people to drive I knew immediately whether my pupils had passed or failed their driving test by the way they got out of the car afterwards.

What we are thinking and feeling will directly affect the way we sit stand and move. Similarly, if we become more conscious of the way we do things and pay attention to what we are doing in every action, even sweeping the floor or washing the dishes can be a consciousness act – and consciousness brings happiness.

PHYSICAL, MENTAL AND EMOTIONAL HABITS

Since the whole basis of the Alexander Technique rests on the principle that it is impossible to separate the physical, mental and emotional processes in any form of human activity, it follows that any physical habits we may have adopted throughout the course of our lives will invariably be present in our mind and emotions. If by being more conscious we are able to change the way that we perform our physical activities, it naturally follows that our mental attitude to life and how we feel emotionally will also change.

It also follows, then, that feelings of unhappiness or being unfulfilled must directly affect the way we use our physical bodies, and this is why Alexander always referred to the 'use of the self' and not to the 'use of the body'. By applying the principles of the Technique (inhibition and direction) we can alter the way in which we think and feel.

Alexander devotes a whole chapter in his book *Constructive Conscious Control of the Individual* to the subject of happiness, in which he writes:

> I shall now endeavour to show that the lack of real happiness manifested by the majority of adults of today is due to the fact that they are experiencing, not an improving, but a continually deteriorating use of their psycho-physical selves. This is associated with those defects, imperfections, undesirable traits of character, disposition, temperament, etc, characteristic of imperfectly co-ordinated people struggling through life beset with certain maladjustments of the psycho-physical organism, which are actually setting up conditions of irritation and pressure during both sleeping and waking hours. Whilst the maladjustments remain present, these malconditions increase day by day and week by week, and foster that unsatisfactory psycho-physical state which we call 'unhappiness'. Small wonder that under these conditions the person concerned becomes more and more irritated and unhappy. Irritation is not compatible with happiness, yet the human creature has to employ this already irritated organism in all the psycho-physical activities demanded by a civilized mode of life. It stands to reason that every effort made by the human creature whose organism is already in an irritated condition must tend to make the creature still more irritated, and therefore as time goes on, his chances of happiness diminish. Furthermore, his

experiences of happiness become of ever shorter duration, until at last he is forced to take refuge in a state of unhappiness, a psycho-physical condition as perverted as that state of ill-health which people reach when they experience a perverted form of satisfaction in the suffering of pain.

The psycho-physical condition of the person afflicted with irritation and pressure is such that all his efforts in any direction will be more or less a failure as compared with the efforts of those who are not so afflicted, and there is probably no stimulus from without which makes more for irritability of the person concerned than failure (either comparative or complete) in accomplishment, nothing which can have a worse effect upon our emotions, self-respect, happiness or confidence – in fact, upon our temperament and character in general.

By changing the way we perform everyday actions we can directly influence the way we think and feel. If we take our time as we perform tasks in a conscious manner we can find that we are enjoying the way we do it. We will naturally feel happier and our minds will be calmer.

In short, the habitual way of being that most of us have been encouraged to adopt from childhood onwards is bound to affect our physical and mental wellbeing. This, in turn, will affect our functioning in a detrimental way, which can cause frustration, anger and lack of confidence or a general state of unhappiness. Then these emotional states will themselves start to become habits (see the diagram opposite).

No one starts out in life feeling angry or frustrated, or starts out in life lacking in confidence or self-worth. These are feelings that we acquire throughout our lives and are not inherent in our mental or emotional make-up.

EXPERIENCES AFFECT OUR MUSCLES

All emotional or mental experiences, whether negative or positive, affect the muscles. If these experiences are stressful and frequent enough, then the muscles learn to stay in a state of tension which eventually becomes fixed within the body. A good example of this is somebody who suffers from depression. Although it is a mental illness, you can actually see the physical depression in their posture. The word 'depression' actually describes a physical shape; after all,

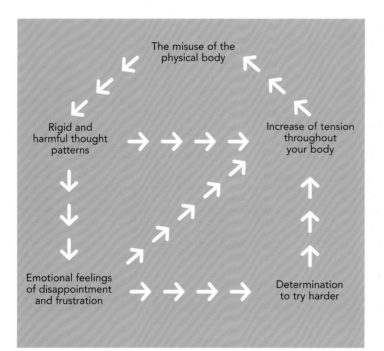

← The perpetual cycle of mental, emotional and physical disharmony.

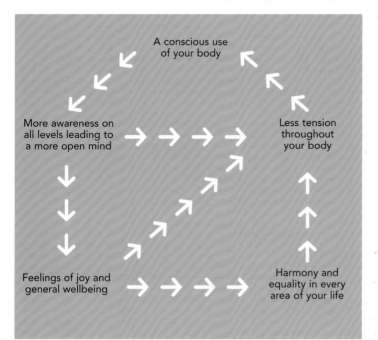

← The perpetual cycle of mental, emotional and physical harmony and wellbeing.

you can depress a cardboard box. So depression is the shape of the body as well as a mental condition. By releasing muscular tension through the application of the Alexander Technique, not only will a person's shape change, so too will their mental outlook on life.

Alexander once said that we translate everything – whether physical, mental or spiritual – into muscular tension. Releasing these muscle tensions can sometimes bring buried emotions to the surface, but do not be concerned as this is quite normal and will soon pass. It is much better, in my opinion, to have these unconscious tensions released rather than being fixed within the body, causing us to behave in a detrimental way both toward ourselves and toward others. Sometimes, when counselling a client, a psychotherapist can make a certain amount of progress with the client and then seem not to get any further. This can be due to the fact that, although the client

exercise

CHANGING YOUR THINKING

1 Lie on the floor with your eyes closed.

2 Think of being in a stressful situation, such as being late for work or perhaps being lost in a strange country with unfriendly people around.

3 After a few minutes, see if you can feel a change in muscle tension.

4 Be aware of your breathing and heartbeat

Now repeat this exercise slightly differently:

1 Again, lie on the floor with your eyes closed.

2 This time, think of relaxing on a beach or in your garden on a beautiful summer's day. Imagine that you are feeling content and everything feels perfect.

3 After a few minutes see if you can feel a difference in muscle tension.

4 Is your breathing and heartbeat different than before?

Remember, it is only your thinking that has changed, but your thinking has probably affected your physical and emotional states.

Patrick's story

Patrick Stanton
Age: 35 | Occupation: builder

Patrick had fallen off a ladder nearly two years previously and had been off work for much of that time. Although his initial injury had healed in a short time, he had been left with a pain in his left knee.

'I had been in constant pain, since my accident, for nearly two years when I stumbled across the Alexander Technique. I had become withdrawn and at times very depressed, which, of course, had repercussions on my family. They were very sympathetic, but after a while the tension began to build, with ever-increasing rows. I couldn't go back to work although I had tried several times and socializing was no fun at all. The pain and torment were beginning to take over my life.

After my fourth or fifth lesson I was able to see that it was I who was causing myself the discomfort. I had got into the habit of tensing up my left leg, which I probably did initially just after I had my accident. I couldn't believe it at first that the problem was so simple; in fact I walked out of that lesson without any pain at all for the first time in 20 months. The pain did, in fact, return the next day, but this experience had given me hope, so I persevered with the lessons and now I am free of the pain for at least 95 per cent of the time. During the process, however, I have learnt so much about myself that I would never have known otherwise. I am deeply grateful to the Technique and to my teacher for the patience that he had.

is looking at mental and emotional issues, he or she is not addressing the state of the body at the same time. Unless the muscular tension is released along with looking at mental and emotional issues, progress can often be limited. A combination of psychotherapy and Alexander Technique can often work very well together.

It is important, however, that the person releases the tension themselves and learns ways of avoiding tension in the future, otherwise the change may well be short-lived. It is essential that the person themselves becomes empowered to change their life.

It is often the case that a person approaches me for Alexander lessons because of physical problems, such as a back or neck problem, yet they often say that they feel calmer and happier as a result of the lessons. Others report that they are sleeping better and arguments within their family home have diminished, while others are surprised because their confidence and self-esteem have increased. With the Alexander Technique you do not have to go back in time to understand or experience past traumas. Releasing tension in the present will help you to improve many aspects of your life.

3

How to Help Yourself

11

Awareness and Observation

We don't see things as they are,
we see things as we are.

ANAÏS NIN, *THE DIARY OF ANAÏS NIN*

It is essential to point out that this book is not a substitute for lessons in the Alexander Technique. As I have said before, a 'teach yourself to drive' book would not preclude the need for driving lessons. It should be used as a helpful guide prior to, or in conjunction with, actual Alexander Technique lessons (see pages 148–153).

The main reason for this is that it is much easier for a person who is objective and experienced in this field to see clearly the 'misuse' of his or her pupil. Remember, it took Alexander a great many hours over several years to discover what caused him to lose his voice. Most of us have neither the time nor the patience to achieve what he did; nor is it necessary. He left behind enough information to make the process of self-discovery far easier, but it is still advisable to have a guide, for the path has numerous pitfalls and obstacles along the way.

It is worth reiterating that we are not learning anything new; this is a process of unlearning. Once we stop doing what is causing the problem, the 'right thing' will automatically take its place.

OBSERVING

Observation of ourselves and others is the first major step to becoming aware of how much we misuse our bodies in even the simplest of activities. It is much easier to see it in others at first, simply because you are more objective. When observing other people try to study the whole of them rather than specific parts, and ask yourself the following questions:

Is this person
- Standing up straight?
- Leaning forward?
- Leaning backward?

If they are leaning forward or backward, where are they bending from?
- From the ankles?
- From the hips?
- From the upper back or shoulders?

A side view may be the best way of seeing clearly an unsymmetrical or misshapen form that so many of us have. You will often notice two or more different tendencies with opposing forces: for example,

someone may be leaning back from their waist while their head
and shoulders are thrown forward from the upper part of the chest
(as in the photograph on the right). It is also interesting to watch
the differing postures that people adopt while they are sitting. If
possible, notice the varying shapes that individuals adopt as life's
internal and external pressures take their toll.

When you start to acquire a sense of the lack of poise in many
of the people you see, begin to observe yourself to see whether you
are doing the same thing. It is essential that you remain as objective
as possible and it helps to have a sense of humour! Alexander used
to say, 'This work is far too serious to be taken seriously.'

If you do notice anything about yourself that you think could
be improved, it is important not to try to bring about a change
immediately. Anything you *do* to improve the situation will

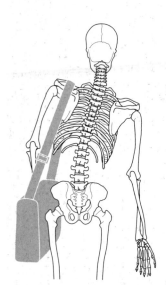
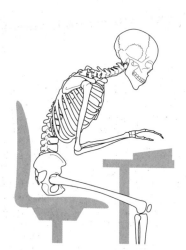

↑ Unbalanced posture can
put a strain on our entire
skeletal system, as well as
on all the internal organs.

↑ A common standing position.
This woman is throwing her
pelvis forward, arching her back
and leaning back from the waist.
In turn, this will cause the legs
to tighten and the shoulders to
hunch forward.

invariably cause an increase in tension, thus encouraging the habit to become more ingrained. It is a common human tendency to bring about the end we desire straightaway, but it is vital to use our reasoning and work out first what is causing the problem. In other words, we have to 'undo' something rather than 'do' something else, and this is easier said than done. This is when Alexander lessons can be invaluable; your teacher will spot immediately when tension in your body is being increased rather than decreased.

Alan's story

Alan Capel
Age: 39 | Occupation: lorry driver

I drive a truck for a living and am completely hooked on surfing. A few years ago a 'nuisance' pain behind my right knee turned into chronic sciatica which caused a pain that stretched from the base of my lumbar spine right down to my toes. This caused my toes to curl under my foot making it difficult and painful to walk and, more importantly, I was unable to drive the truck.

Being a surfer I was an optimist, and I wasn't insured for such an event. My whole life ethic of 'work hard, play hard' was suddenly thrown back in my face, and I did not know why. All the people I turned to for help did not know either.

No work... let alone surfing. No football. No achievement. No pride. No satisfaction. No fulfilment. No justification for the pain – just the endless throbbing, which was robbing me of my life energy.

My eldest son, then three years old, did not understand why his dad could not rough and tumble with him and, with the arrival of his younger brother, I was desperately seeking the answer to my problem. Within six weeks of the birth of my younger son, I was in hospital for the removal of a prolapsed intervertebral disc pressing on the sciatic nerve at the base of my spine. Two weeks later I was back at home in a worse state than ever, having been told by my surgeon that my discs were fine. While there was no doubt in the consultant's mind that I was in considerable pain, he could offer me no explanation for the cause.

Doctors, osteopaths, physiotherapists, acupuncturists, consultants, nurses, surgeons and even faith healers had all done their best, but to no avail... It was at this point that a friend recommended a course of lessons in the Alexander Technique.

I started having lessons mainly because I could not think of what else to do. There were no overnight miracles, but I was not expecting any. After 15 lessons real changes started to happen; changes that not only led to a reduction in pain, but changes on levels that I never knew existed. Make no mistake, the Alexander Technique belongs in the realms of re-education in how you use both your body and your mind. The Technique has given me the opportunity to lose some of the harmful habits that were at the root of my sciatica, and has enabled me to get back into the driving seat of my own life. Real free choice is back in my hands once again.

STANDING

To become more aware of yourself while standing, ask the following questions:

- Am I standing more on one leg than the other, or am I equally balanced on both of my legs? Even if you are equally balanced, try moving over so that there is slightly more weight on one leg than the other, then reverse the process. Whichever position feels more comfortable will indicate your habit.
- Am I standing more on my heels or more on the balls of my feet? This will help to indicate whether you are leaning backward or forward.
- Am I standing more on the outside or on the inside of my feet? Note: this can be different for each foot; for example, you may be standing on the outside of the left foot and on the inside of the right.
- Are my knees locked back with excess tension or are they over-relaxed so that my knees are bent?

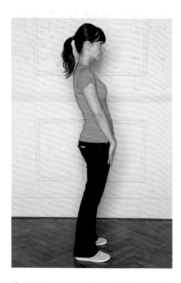 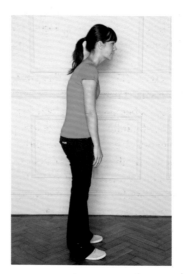 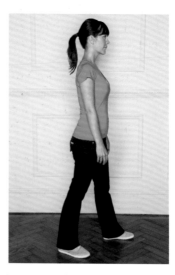

↑ This woman is not balanced. She is leaning backward, causing an over-arching of her back, which is likely to lead to lower back problems.

↑ This time she is leaning too far forward, which can be the result of spending many hours slumped over a desk.

↑ Now she is poised and balanced and the muscular system is required to do far less.

Any other aspects of standing will involve our sense of proprioception (the sense that tells us where we are in space), which may be extremely unreliable; it is therefore necessary to use either a mirror or a video camera to obtain accurate information.

If, by asking any of the previous questions, you begin to notice you have a habit of standing in an unbalanced way, it is helpful to exaggerate the tendency for a short while to get a sense of how much strain this habit is causing throughout your whole structure. In other words, if you are inclined to stand more on your left leg and on the outside of your feet, then exaggerate this habit still further, so as to stand even more on to your left side and more on the outside of your feet. Within a few moments you can begin to get a sense of your whole structure being out of balance. This feeling is always with us to a certain extent, but we are unaware of it because our habit overrides our sense of proprioception.

Simply by being conscious of the way we stand can start to bring about a change that is desirable for our wellbeing.

IMPROVING YOUR STANDING POSITION

Although Alexander did not advocate a correct way of standing, as this would encourage a new set of habits, he did leave behind a few useful suggestions to remember while standing:

- Place the feet at approximately 30 cm (12 in) apart. This gives a more solid base to support the rest of the body.
- When standing for long periods, it is helpful to place one foot approximately 15 cm (6 in) behind the other, with the weight of the body resting chiefly on the rear foot. The feet should be making a 45 degree angle to each other. This prevents sinking down into one hip, which can affect the balance of the whole structure. This is particularly helpful to those of us who have a habit of standing more on one leg than the other.
- If you notice that you are pushing your pelvis forward, allow it to go back without altering the balance and without deliberately throwing the body forward. This helps to eliminate the very common tendency of pushing the pelvis forward when in a standing position. It is best to use a long mirror side-on when doing this observation exercise.
- There are three points on each foot which form a tripod. The first point is the heel, the second is the ball, and the third is

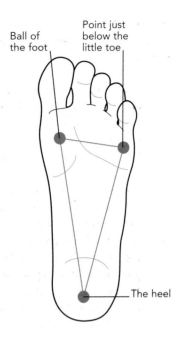

Ball of the foot

Point just below the little toe

The heel

↑ **The sole of the foot showing the three points that should be in contact with the ground in order to set up a tripod effect, which helps us to keep our balance.**

situated at the beginning of the little toe (see the illustration on page 127). It is well known by engineers that an object needs at least three points of contact to be stable. So, if we are only standing on two of the three points, we will be less balanced and consequently many more muscles will be tense, trying to maintain the body's equilibrium. Next time your shoes wear out, have a look at where they are worn down most, as this will give a good indication about whether or not there is even pressure throughout the whole foot.

exercise

STANDING BEFORE A MIRROR

Use a mirror or even two when doing this exercise:

1 Stand with your eyes closed, facing the mirror in a way that feels comfortable.

2 Open your eyes and see if your idea of how you were standing matches the reality.

3 With your eyes still closed, try to align yourself in front of the mirror so that you feel completely symmetrical.

4 Open your eyes once again, to see if what you see and what you are feeling match.

5 Repeat the above while standing sideways to the mirror.

SITTING

In a similar way to how you observed yourself in the standing exercise, you can ask the following questions while sitting:

- Am I sitting squarely on both of my sitting bones, or do I prefer to sit more to one side?
- Do I usually cross my legs while sitting and, if so, do I have a preference as to which leg I cross?
- Am I slumped while sitting or do I have a tendency to sit up in a rigid fashion?

designers really understand the mechanics of the human body. Therefore, if you do have to sit for hours on end, make sure you get up and walk around every so often. There may also be times when you could walk to nearby places instead of using the car.

It is worth noting that the spine is under much more stress when sitting than when standing. Most chairs, especially car seats, slope backward, encouraging the person sitting on them to slump forward, and the person has to tense many muscles to counteract this effect. You can, however, buy chairs that have an adjustable seat so that you can have it flat or sloping forward when needed. This helps to prevent the slumping or the sinking down into the hips that so often occurs. You can produce the same effect by placing a 5-cm (2-in) piece of wood or a couple of telephone books under the back legs of any chair. Try it for yourself.

A cost-effective solution is to place a wedge-shaped cushion on most chairs that slope backward. Information on where to find wedge-shaped cushions and supportive chairs can be found on page 155.

↓ 1. A chair with a sloping base tends to encourage poor posture.
2. Try putting books under the back legs of a chair and see how different it feels.

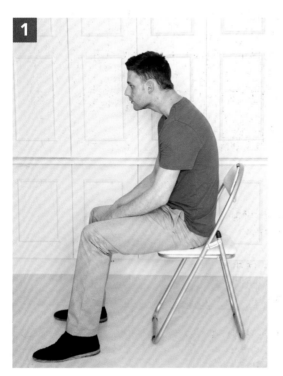

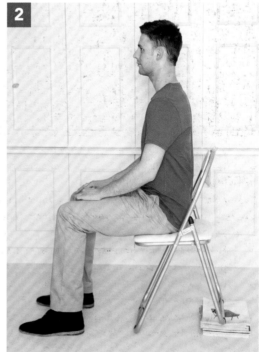

Give Your Back a Rest

A perfect spine is an all-important factor in preserving those conditions and uses of the human machine which work together for perfect health, yet there are comparatively few people who do not in some form or degree suffer, perhaps quite unconsciously, from spinal curvature.

FREDERICK MATTHIAS ALEXANDER

Back pain is rife in our society. According to latest figures published by the The Health and Safety Executive, back pain will affect as many as four out of five people in Britain. In the US, the statistics are no better – according to the Bureau of Labor, American citizens spend a staggering $15 billion per year on medical care and disability payments due to back pain. As a health problem, back pain is the third most expensive disorder after heart disease and cancer.

Over the years there has been little research into the Alexander Technique, but one major study was run in the UK by Southampton and Bristol Universities. Its findings, published in the *British Medical Journal* in August 2008, make interesting reading.

The results show that those who had a course of Alexander lessons reported an overall beneficial effect on back pain, significantly decreasing days in pain and improving the functioning and quality of life of patients. This research trial compared the long-term benefits for the following groups: those who had six lessons in the Alexander Technique, those who had 24 lessons in the Technique, those who had six sessions of a classic massage and those who undertook doctor-prescribed aerobic exercise.

The best results were seen in the group that had 24 lessons in the Alexander Technique, with important improvements in function, quality of life and reduction in days in pain. People who had had Alexander lessons reported continual improvements a year after they stopped the lessons.

Before we discuss how to help back pain, it might be helpful to first understand how the spine functions.

THE SPINE

The spine, also known as the vertebral column or the backbone, forms an essential part of the skeleton. It acts both as a pillar which supports the upper parts of the body and as a protection to the spinal cord and the nerves which arise from it. The spinal column is built up of a number of bones placed one upon another; these are called the vertebrae. The presence of a spinal cord which is supported by a vertebral column in more evolved types of animal gives them the title of 'vertebrates' and, of all the vertebrates, it is only man who can stand absolutely erect. This, besides having distinct advantages, brings with it certain problems – the main one being that gravity is now bearing down upon a structure that is extremely unstable because it has two legs instead of four.

The spine is about 70 cm (28 in) long in a fully grown adult. Differences in height mainly depend upon the length of the lower limbs. There are 33 vertebrae which make up the complete spinal column, although in adults five of these are fused together to form the sacrum, and a further four to form the coccyx; the actual number of separate bones is therefore reduced to 26. Of these, there are seven in the neck area which are referred to as the cervical vertebrae; 12 below these which all have ribs attached and are known as the thoracic or dorsal vertebrae; a further five below these which are called the lumbar vertebrae and, lastly, the nine which go to make up the sacrum and coccyx.

An important feature of the spine, especially marked in human beings, is the presence of four curves. These curves strengthen the structure so that it can bear more weight, and they also act as a spring to minimize any jolting or jarring of the internal organs. If the curves become too straight or, more often, too pronounced, the spine will lose some of these properties. That is, it will become weaker and will not suspend and support the organs as efficiently as it should. It is also very important to realize that these curves can change depending on the activity that is being performed. For example, have a look at the back of a child who is squatting or sitting and you will find that the lower back looks very straight. When medical people talk about the curves always having been present, they are often referring to the inside of the spine and you can see this only in an x-ray or MRI scan.

Cervical curviture

Thoracic curviture

Lumbar curviture

Sacral curviture

↑ Diagram of the spine showing the four different curves while standing.

INTERVERTEBRAL DISCS

Between each vertebra lies a thick layer of fibro-cartilage known as the intervertebral disc. Each disc consists of an outer portion, which is known as the annulus fibrosus, and an inner core known as the nucleus pulposus.

The annulus fibrosus

This part of the disc is made up of concentric fibres which keep the nucleus in place when it is under pressure from above.

The nucleus pulposus

This central part of the disc consists of a gelatinous substance which is transparent. It is in fact made up of 88 per cent water, and it is this nucleus that takes the brunt of the body's weight (see the illustration above).

column and found that the ratio between the thickness of the discs and the thickness of the adjacent vertebrae diminished with age:

- At birth they were the same size.
- At the age of 10, the disc was half the size of the vertebra.
- At 24, the disc was a third of the size of the vertebra.
- At 60, the disc was a quarter of the size of the vertebra.

Up to the age of 20, the bones are still growing so some of these figures are not surprising. But, after the early 20s, there is no reason for the discs to diminish in size apart from the excess pressure that is placed on them by continuous muscular tension. This pressure causes a gradual loss of fluid from the fibro-cartilage of which the discs are largely composed. The spine is a hydraulic system which works by absorbing and releasing water; a healthy disc can in fact absorb up to 20 times its volume of water. You can see that if the discs have shrunk in size then the spine cannot work to its maximum capability.

If you lie down regularly each day for a mere 20 minutes, not only are you easing or preventing backache, but you will be ensuring that the discs in your back are able to maintain their correct shape for longer. This will give you the chance to move in a more effortless way.

The way in which you go into and come out of the semi-supine position is also very important. The photographs below and overleaf will help you to get the most out of your session.

↘ **Find a suitable area to lie down. Take the correct number of books with you.**

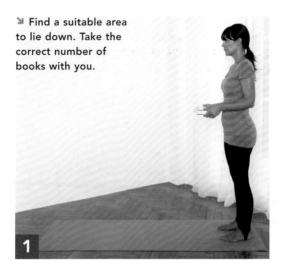

↘ **While thinking of your directions, put one leg forward and go down on one knee.**

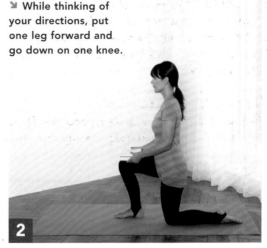

⭢ Place the books to your right or left, roughly where your head will be when you are lying down.

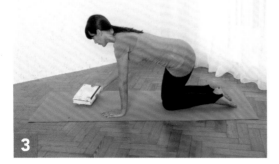

⭢ Place your hands on the ground so that you are on all fours.

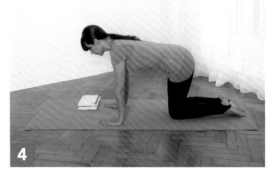

⭢ Balance on your hands and toes and lower your legs to the ground with your knees pointing away from the books.

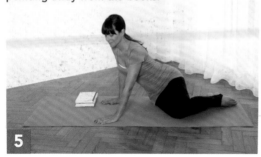

⭢ Bring your right hand through between your left hand and your knee.

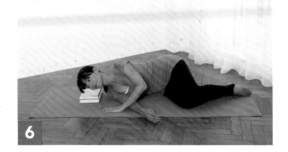

⭢ Gently roll over onto your back, adjusting the position of the books so that they are comfortably under the back of your head.

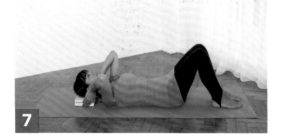

⭢ Bring your knees upward, positioning your feet so that they are as near as possible to your torso while still remaining comfortable.

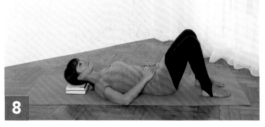

❯ Decide which way you wish to get up. Look in that direction and then let your head gently roll the same way.

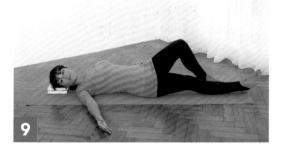

9

❯ Let your whole body roll in the same direction as the head.

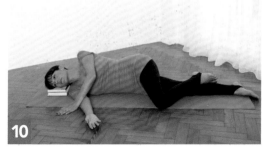

10

❯ Roll over on to your front with the support of a hand and a leg.

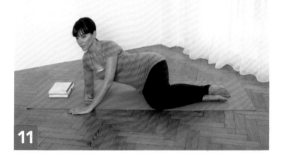

11

❯ Raise yourself until you are on all fours once again.

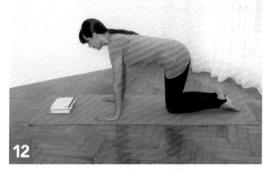

12

❯ Pick up the books and then place one leg in front of the other.

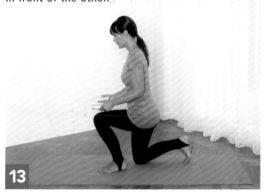

13

❯ Thinking of the head going forward and up, lean forward and you will naturally come back to the standing position.

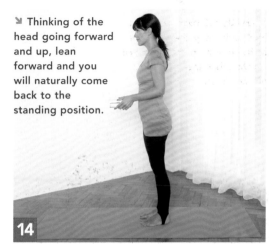

14

13

Improve Your Breathing Naturally

The same stream of life that runs through my veins night and day runs through the world and dances in rhythmic measures.

It is the same life that shouts in joy through the dust of the Earth in numberless blades of grass and breaks into tumultuous waves of leaves and flowers.

It is the same life that rocked in the ocean cradle of birth and of death, in ebb and in flow.

I feel my limbs are made glorious by the touch of this world of life and my pride is from life, the throb of ages dancing in my blood this moment.

RABINDRANATH TAGORE, FROM *GITANJALI*

Without our breath nothing else would have any importance whatsoever. In fact, we would not even exist. Our breath is our number one priority, for without it we are unable to utter one single word or perform even the smallest of actions. The life force itself automatically causes us to take a breath without any effort on our part; we do not even have to remember to breathe as it all happens by reflex. Saint Augustine once said that people travel to wonder at the heights of mountains, at the huge waves of the sea, at the long courses of rivers, at the vast compass of the ocean, at the circular motion of the stars and, all too often, they pass by themselves without wondering. Perhaps it would be good from time to time to wonder at the power that is behind the breath.

exercise

BE AWARE OF YOUR BREATHING

Just pause for a moment as you are reading these words to become aware of that silent inhalation and exhalation which is with you every moment of your life. Without it, you would not be able to see these words, hear the sound of the pages as they turn, feel the texture of the paper, or even move one muscle to hold this book. Contemplate the mysteries of your breath and see if you can get a sense of what is the force or energy that is drawing the air into and then out of your lungs.

POSTURE AND BREATHING

Efficient and beneficial breathing is an integral part of good posture, a clear mind and using your body in the way it was designed to be used. Like many other functions of the body, this simple act of breathing is often unconsciously interfered with. As we have seen, poor posture and misuse of the body can cause an over-tensing of the entire muscular system. This can affect the functioning of the rib-cage, the lungs and even the nasal passage, mouth and throat (trachea) through which the air passes. Muscle tension can also produce a general 'collapsing', or pulling down, of the whole upper body, which can result in a considerable limitation in the lungs' capacity to take in air. This can lead to shallow breathing, causing us to make an extra effort just to have sufficient air. In short, we can make the effortless act of breathing very hard work. This extra exertion goes largely unnoticed because we become accustomed to our shallow and strained breathing. This is the way we have breathed for many years and therefore it will feel 'normal' and 'right' to us.

This start of the interference with the respiratory system can often be traced back to around the age of five or six because of the posture we had to adopt when bending over school desks. We are forced to hold these 'set' positions for a great many hours during most of our developing years, and the poor posture which subsequently develops causes ungraceful, unco-ordinated or even clumsy movements and restricted breathing patterns. If your body is unable to get enough oxygen because its natural deeper breathing is being interfered with, it will have to find another way of achieving this objective in order to get the oxygen it requires. The breathing rate will need to increase and, as a result, a quicker, shallower type of respiration occurs and in this way we start to develop habitual ways of breathing.

When Alexander first began teaching his Technique, he was nicknamed: 'The Breathing Man'. This was because, initially, he developed his technique to help people breathe in a better way. Most of his pupils were suffering with voice strain, asthma or just shallow breathing. After a lesson, his pupils noticed a remarkable difference in their breathing as they started to release the muscular tension that was interfering with their natural breathing.

BREATHING EXERCISES

Many voice trainers and physical educators encourage 'deep breathing' as a way of getting the lungs to work as they should and, while their aim may be sound in principle, the way they encourage their students to achieve this may actually exacerbate many respiratory problems. People are often instructed to increase their lung capacity by 'pulling in' or 'pushing out' their breath, but this only adds further tension to an already over-strained muscular system. Almost all breathing exercises focus on the in-breath, as in, for example, the instruction to 'take a deep breath', but this will invariably cause the person to interfere with the breathing mechanisms even further. Tightening and shortening the muscles can result in the person arching their back and lifting the chest, which actually restricts the breathing even further, causing additional detrimental breathing patterns or ingraining the original breathing habits even more deeply.

Like the rest of the Alexander Technique, breathing naturally is a process of *unlearning* detrimental habits, rather than practising certain breathing exercises or techniques. Dr Wilfred Barlow was convinced that the asthmatic needed 'breathing education' rather than a set of exercises. In his book *The Alexander Principle,* he says:

> Breathing exercises have, of course, frequently been given by physiotherapists for this (asthma) and for other breathing conditions, but the fact is that breathing exercises do not help the asthmatic greatly – in fact, recent studies show that after a course of 'breathing exercises', the majority of people breathe less efficiently than they did before they started them.

IMPROVING BREATHING

Alexander was a trained actor, and efficient breathing was essential to his skilful recitation. His Technique involved becoming aware and preventing poor breathing habits. It is based on *'doing less'* and one of his most famous quotations was 'I see at last that if I don't breathe... I breathe'.

Many performing actors, singers and even teachers find the Technique dramatically helps their breathing and helps them to achieve an improved voice production without strain. By ensuring that we breathe naturally, we can also effectively combat the effects of stress that often comes with public speaking. In this way, we can feel calmer and more in control even at times of intense emotional or mental stress.

Contrary to what many people think, it is the out-breath, rather than the in-breath, that determines the way we breathe. As we exhale the atmospheric pressure in our lungs decreases, creating a partial vacuum which causes the air from outside to be sucked into our lungs *without us having to do anything.* Under normal conditions, the entire breathing mechanism should be self-governing and therefore is sometimes referred to as working 'autonomically'. The more carbon dioxide we exhale, the deeper the next inhalation will be and the deeper our breathing will become.

exercise

BECOME AWARE OF THE BREATH

Take a moment to lie down in the semi-supine position as described on page 136 and begin to be aware of your breathing. It is often easier to detect tension in this position. Ask yourself the following questions:

- How rapid is my breathing?
- How deeply do I breathe?
- Are my ribs moving as I breathe?
- How much movement is there in the abdominal region when I breathe?
- How much movement is there throughout the rib-cage when I breathe?
- Is the movement of my breath evenly on the left and right side of the ribs?
- Do I feel any restriction in my breathing and, if so, where?

It is vital that you do not deliberately change the way you breathe. Simply bringing your awareness to the inhalation and the exhalation of your breath may be enough to bring about a favourable change. Just by spending a few minutes observing any restriction in and around the rib-cage and abdominal area, you can start to breathe more naturally.

To help his pupils re-learn breathing naturally, Alexander developed 'the whispered ah procedure'. He maintained that he did not like using exercises, as they could encourage habits and stop people thinking for themselves, but he made an exception for the 'whispered ah' exercise because he said that it was essentially an exercise in inhibition and its aim was to prevent 'end-gaining' while breathing.

Regular practise of the 'whispered ah' will help you to notice detrimental breathing habits and develop a more efficient respiratory system. Once again, it is strongly recommended that initially you go through this routine with your Alexander teacher, as it is easy to misinterpret the instructions. This is because most of us suffer from what Alexander referred to as Faulty Sensory Appreciation, which simply means that, even when we are following instructions to the best of our ability, we may be doing something else entirely without realizing it. For example, it is very common for people to pull their head back rather than let the jaw drop while carrying out Step 3 (see exercise on page 147), while others are convinced that they are opening their mouth wide when there is actually less than 2 cm (1 in)

exercise

THE 'WHISPERED AH PROCEDURE'

1 First notice where your tongue is, and let it rest on the floor of the mouth with the tip lightly touching your lower front teeth. This allows for a free passage of air to and from the lungs.

2 Make sure your lips and facial muscles are not tense. To assist in this, it may be helpful to think of something that makes you smile.

3 Gently and without straining, let your lower jaw drop so that your mouth is open. If you allow gravity to do most of the work you will make sure that your head does not tilt backward in the process.

4 Whisper an 'ah' sound (as in the word 'father') until you come to the natural end of the breath. It is important not to rush the procedure by forcing the air out too quickly or by trying to empty the lungs by extending the 'ah' sound as long as possible.

5 Gently close your lips and allow the air to come in through your nose and fill up your lungs.

6 Repeat this procedure several times.

between their upper and lower lips. If, for any reason, you are unable to have lessons, it is advisable to perform the 'whispered ah' in front of a mirror, as this will give you some idea of whether or not you are carrying out the instructions correctly.

It is essential to understand that the respiratory mechanism works by reflex, and is therefore completely automatic. Anything we do in order to improve our breathing will only interfere with it further. We need to 'get out of the way' and let nature take its course.

THE ENJOYMENT OF BREATHING

Breathing is not only an essential part of existence, but it can be one of life's great joys. It can be a pure pleasure to feel the air filling you and offering you the gift of yet another moment to appreciate life's wonders. Being aware of your breathing and practising the 'whispered ah' regularly can powerfully eliminate the effects of stress, as it calms your entire system and allows you to return to the present moment to experience the true miracle of being alive.

What to Expect in an Alexander Lesson

All I need to say in this place is that I am sure, as a matter of personal experience and observation, that it gives all the things we have been looking for in a system of physical education: relief from strain due to maladjustment, and consequent improvement in physical and mental health; increased consciousness of the physical means employed to gain the end proposed by the will and, along with this a general heightening of consciousness on all levels; a technique of inhibition, working on the physical level to prevent the body from slipping back, under the influence of greedy 'end-gaining', into its old habits of mal-coordination, and working to inhibit undesirable impulses and irrelevance on the emotional and intellectual levels respectively. We cannot ask more from any system of physical education; nor if we seriously desire to alter human beings in a desirable direction, can we ask any less?

ALDOUS HUXLEY, *ENDS AND MEANS*

INDIVIDUAL LESSONS

This is clearly the best way to find out more about yourself and the harmful habits that you have. A lesson will usually last between 30 and 45 minutes, and the aims of the lessons are:

- To detect any tension that you may be holding unnecessarily and then to release it.
- To become aware of the habits of mind-body use that are causing the tension, and to change these if you so wish.
- To develop different ways of performing actions which will not create so much tension in the first place.
- To teach you inhibition and apply directions.
- To give you an experience of an improved use of yourself.

THE ROLE OF THE TEACHER

The teacher's role is to point out your own personal habits and to explain why they are so harmful. They will give certain directions to help you combat your old ways of moving through verbal instructions and by using hands, much of which is carried out around the head, neck and back area. The touch of the hands is very subtle, and will not aggravate any pain. However, if you are suffering a great deal of pain it may be advisable to obtain treatment (from your doctor, chiropractor or osteopath) before going for lessons.

The teacher may also work with you on a table at first. (Note: you will not be required to remove your clothes – except perhaps your shoes.) In this position, your body is more stable and therefore it can be much easier for you to release muscle tension.

You may be taken through a series of movements, such as sitting or walking, so that you can learn different ways of moving. If any of these activities cause you discomfort or pain, your teacher will be happy to review these with you to shed light on the cause. Occasionally, you may experience an extra ache or tension; this should not last for more than a few hours, and is probably due to the fact that those muscles have previously been underused. An Alexander lesson can also be applied to almost any activity, including playing sport or a musical instrument.

The number of lessons needed can vary from person to person, but the changes will often be noticeable after the first lesson. These changes may be short-lived to begin with, but the effects will remain for longer periods after more lessons.

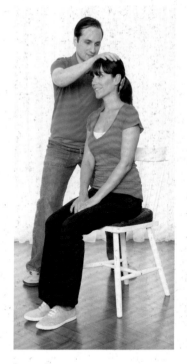

↑ An Alexander teacher works with a pupil to release tension and achieve a free, dynamic relationship of the head, neck and upper back.

The price of lessons varies a great deal, depending on the location and experience of the teacher. Some people are put off by the price of a course, but it is worth considering that the cost is less than that of an average holiday and the effects will last long after a holiday is only a distant memory. It is a matter of priorities; this could be essential for your future wellbeing. If you really cannot afford a full course of lessons then even a few will definitely help, but you should discuss this with your teacher before you start.

I strongly recommended you try one lesson from a variety of teachers before embarking on a series of lessons, because a good rapport will greatly enhance the process of change. When choosing a teacher you must make sure they have undertaken a three-year full-time training programme of not less than 1,600 hours.

There is a list of all the Alexander Technique societies throughout the world on pages 155–156.

LEARNING IN GROUPS

It can also be of great value to participate in group classes. These are often organized by local adult education authorities. Even if you are already having private lessons, group sessions can be very revealing. It is easier to perceive misuse in someone else when they are performing simple acts like walking, standing or sitting, and many of us share the same habits. Watching other people can help you to make comparisons and may give you a better idea of what you are doing. You then have the choice of whether or not to change your unconscious behaviour patterns. Although a group session is not as beneficial as an individual lesson, I have still been amazed at the physical changes in people who come to these classes and by the noticeable difference in their outlook on life.

Whether you have private lessons or learn in a group situation, I reiterate my point that your current habits will *feel right* and a new use of yourself is therefore bound to feel very alien. This feeling is only temporary. Within a few weeks, the new way of moving will begin to feel natural and your old habits will feel clumsy and awkward. You have to approach it with the idea of *unlearning*, rather than learning something new.

You must be prepared to be told where you are going wrong, and this is something none of us likes. The irony is that, as we progress, we will be improving our use of ourselves but we will often not know it.

Patsy's story

Patsy Spiers
Age: 49 | Occupation: midwife

Patsy started coming to a class with 12 others. She was suffering from a stiff neck that gave her pain whenever she turned her head. She was also prone to frequent and severe migraine headaches and she had a wheezy chest that had led to her first asthma attack and greatly worried her. After attending the class for two terms, including a little individual work, she reported:

'The Alexander Technique, which is a way of allowing the body and mind to work together in order to avoid muscular tension, has constantly helped me to be calmer in stressful situations. It has also helped me to be more relaxed while driving. The stiff and painful neck has returned to normal, my wheeziness has improved greatly, with no sign of the asthma returning, and my migraines are far less frequent and not nearly so intense. Although I feel I have a long way to go, I'm a lot more aware of myself so, whenever I get twinges of pain, I adjust accordingly and the pain immediately eases. Although I still suffer from headaches, it takes a lot more physical and mental stress before they manifest.'

The right thing to do would be the last thing we should do, left to ourselves, because it would be the last thing we should think it would be the right thing to do.

The physical, mental and spiritual potentialities of the human being are greater than we have ever realized, greater perhaps than the human mind in its present evolutionary stage is capable of realizing.

We must break the chains which have so held us to that directive mental plane which belongs to the early stages of his evolution. The adoption of conscious guidance and control, which is man's supreme inheritance, must follow, and the outcome will be a race of men and women who will outstrip their ancestors in every known sphere, and enter new spheres as yet undreamt of by the great majority of the civilized peoples of our time.

FREDERICK MATTHIAS ALEXANDER

I will leave you with a quote from Mahatma Gandhi, who said 'It is health that is real wealth and not pieces of gold and silver.' So, really, the question is not whether you can afford to take Alexander lessons, but rather, can you afford not to?

Benefits of a one-to-one lesson

THE PHYSICAL BENEFITS

As you put the principles of the Alexander Technique into practice, any pain you may be feeling due to malco-ordination or excessive tension throughout the muscular system will slowly but surely begin to diminish. The intensity of the pain will start to abate, and the intervals between the bouts of pain will gradually lengthen. This may take some time but, unlike many forms of treatment, the effects of Alexander lessons are often permanent.

It is important to understand, however, that *you* have a definite part to play; the teacher can only help. It is you who has to make the deliberate and reasoned decision to alter your way of being. This is why the Alexander Technique is never heralded as a cure or remedy. The only person who brings about a cure is you yourself – you have only to be taught how to do it.

The effect of a lesson is to experience lightness and ease within your body and a sense of being generally more in touch with your body. This effect will last only a short time at first, but will gradually increase as your lessons progress. Eventually, you will be able to retain this feeling of wellbeing between lessons and it is then that you may reduce the frequency of your lessons.

Many people report sensations of 'floating down the street' or 'walking on air' as movements start to become effortless and people start to move through life with much greater ease.

THE EMOTIONAL BENEFITS

The sensation of physical lightness that we experience has a profound effect on how we feel emotionally. Pupils who have been highly strung or anxious begin to feel calmer; those who have been depressed start to feel brighter and realize that life isn't quite so bad after all. People on the whole begin to feel happier within themselves, which of course rubs off on people around them and consequently has many repercussions in their lives.

It should be remembered, however, that any emotion suppressed for a long time may emerge, and this may be a little uncomfortable for a short while. The most common emotions to be suppressed are anger and sadness, and you may indeed start to experience these at the slightest thing. This is a normal part of the process and will quickly pass. If necessary, discuss any emotional changes with your teacher, for they will be more than happy to reassure you.

Generally, however, it is the positive emotions – happiness, joy, contentment, freedom – that have been repressed and it is these that start to surface. When this happens we can begin to reduce feelings of unhappiness, misery, sadness and gloom from our lives.

THE MENTAL BENEFITS

Because the result of a lesson is to feel much calmer, we will be able to think more clearly about the decisions we have to make in life. We will actually have more time to think about these things and thus be more likely to make the correct choices from day to day. Making the right decisions will naturally make us feel better about ourselves.

Alexander insisted that his Technique was not so much a technique for alleviating physical symptoms, but to 'quicken the conscious mind.' It is as much a method of improving the way we use our minds as it is a way of improving posture. In short, the Technique helps us become more reasonable and clear-thinking human beings; our self-esteem is boosted and our self-confidence improves.

THE SPIRITUAL BENEFITS

When we feel emotionally calmer, mentally more balanced and physically lighter, we can more easily begin to experience our spirit – the joy of existence. Many people have this feeling as a child, but we tend to lose it as we become involved in the superficialities of present-day living. Alexander lessons will help the chains of our rigid thought patterns fall away to reveal a being that we had forgotten existed. We can begin to feel a deep peace and inner freedom… we start to feel who we really are. Alexander called this our 'supreme inheritance'.

Understanding the Terminology

Being present/attentive Being in the present moment and focusing your attention on the activity you are performing. Not letting your mind wander into the past or future.

Conscious control This is the main aim of practising the Alexander Technique. It is a state of being where you are using awareness and free choice to make clear, informed decisions about your actions, rather than reacting in a stereotyped, habitual way.

Direction A mental order that your mind gives to the body.

End-gaining Being too goal-orientated. Thinking only of the end and not giving any consideration to the way that you achieve the goal.

Faulty sensory appreciation Also called faulty sensory perception. Thinking or sensing you are doing one thing when you are doing something completely different. For example, you may feel that you are standing up straight when, in fact, you are leaning backward.

Fear reflex Alexander used this term to describe the body's reaction to any stimulus that causes fear. Any fearful conditions can cause excessive muscular tension which, if happen frequently, can start to develop into a habit. A good example of this is the over-contraction of the neck muscles, which can continuously pull the head back onto the spine causing neck and back problems.

Free choice To become aware of unconscious habits and choose a different reaction to our habitual one.

Habit/habitual actions Any action or thought that we feel is difficult not to do or to think. Often habits are below the level of consciousness and, therefore, we are completely unaware of them.

Inhibition A moment of pausing to give us a chance not to rush into making a decision or into performing an activity without due consideration.

Kinaesthesis/Kinaesthetic sense The sense that informs you where your body is in space at any given time. The brain detects movements of the muscles and senses any movement you are making.

Means whereby Paying attention to the action you are doing, which involves inhibition and direction. Working out in advance how you are going to go about your activity.

Mind-wandering Allowing your thoughts to move away from the present moment. Not paying attention.

Proprioception The sense that tells us where parts of our body are in relation to other parts and in space.

Primary control A dynamic relationship between the head, neck and the rest of the body which helps to harmoniously co-ordinate movement and posture.

Psycho-physical unity The mind and the body act as one unit. They are not separate and each has a powerful influence on the other.

Self The entire human being, including everything mental, physical, emotional and spiritual.

Tension Muscular activity, most of which is totally unnecessary. We obviously need a certain amount of tension, but many people have far too much for a healthy life.

Thinking in activity Using inhibition and direction while performing any action.

Use More than just posture; it the way or ways that we carry out all our activities, including breathing.

Useful Websites

Richard Brennan's websites with useful articles and information about the Alexander Technique
www.alexander.ie
www.alexandertechniqueireland.com

The Alexander Technique Self-Help CD
This is the perfect accompaniment to *The Alexander Technique Workbook* and gives clear and concise instructions on:
How to eliminate unwanted tension, how to prevent or relieve back pain, how to improve your breathing, how to clear your mind of unwanted thoughts, how to practise the two Alexander principles of Inhibition and Direction and how to stay in the present moment.
www.alexander.ie/audio.html

Wedge cushions for cars and chairs
www.alexander.ie/cushion.html

Footwear designed with the Alexander Technique in mind
www.vivobarefoot.com
www.terraplana.com/vivobarefoot_benefits.php

Direction Magazine A wonderful magazine publishing articles and information for teachers and students of the Alexander Technique. Visit the website for free audios, articles, live interviews, plus 25 years of back issues in stock!
www.directionjournal.com

The International Societies of Teachers of the Alexander Technique listed below give details of how to find a teacher nearest to you. All teachers listed on these websites have undergone extensive three-year training.

AUSTRALIA
Australian Society of Teachers of the Alexander Technique (AuSTAT)
www.austat.org.au

BELGIUM
Belgian Association of teachers of the Alexander Technique (AEFMAT)
http://www.fmalexandertech.be

BRAZIL
Associacao Brasileira de Tecnica Alexander (ABTA)
http://abtalexander.com.brr

CANADA
Canadian Society of Teachers of the F. M. Alexander Technique/Société Canadienne des Professeurs de la Technique F. M. Alexander (CANSTAT)
www.canstat.ca

DENMARK
Dansk forening af lærere i Alexanderteknik (DFLAT)
www.dflat.dk

FINLAND
Suomen Alexander-tekniikan Opettajat (FINSTAT)
www.finstat.fi

FRANCE
L'Association Francaise des Professeurs de La Technique Alexander (APTA)
www.techniquealexander.info

GERMANY
Alexander Technik Verband Deutschland (ATVD)
www.alexander-technik.org

IRELAND/EIRE

The Irish Society of Alexander Technique Teachers (ISATT)

www.isatt.ie

www.stat.org.uk

ISRAEL

The Israeli Society of Teachers of the Alexander Technique

www.alexander.org.il

THE NETHERLANDS

Nederlandse Vereniging van Leraren in de Alexander Techniek (NeVLAT)

www.alexandertechniek.nl

NEW ZEALAND

Alexander Technique Teachers' Society of New Zealand (ATTSNZ)

www.alexandertechnique.org.nz

NORWAY

Norsk Forening for Laerere i Alexanderteknikk (NFLAT)

www.alexanderteknikk.no

SOUTH AFRICA

South African Society of Teachers of the Alexander Technique (SASTAT)

www.alexandertechnique.org.za

SPAIN

Spanish Society of Teachers of the Alexander Technique (APTAE)

www.aptae.net

SWITZERLAND

Schweizerischer Verband der Lehrerinnen und Lehrer der F.M. Alexander-Technik (SVLAT/ASPITA)

www.alexandertechnik.ch

UK

This is the website for teachers of the Society of Teachers of the Alexander Technique (STAT), the first and longest-established Alexander Technique organization. Teachers listed are mainly from the UK and Ireland, but also include many other countries.

www.stat.org.uk

UNITED STATES OF AMERICA

American Society for the Alexander Technique (AmSAT)

www.alexandertech.org

Other interesting websites include:

www.alexandertechnique.org

www.alexandertechnique.com

www.ati-net.com

www.atcongress.com

www.alexandertechniqueworldwide.com

www.mouritz.co.uk

www.mtpress.com

www.alexanderbooks.co.uk

www.davidreedmedia.co.uk

www.bodymap.org

www.posturepage.com

Further Reading

Easy to follow and informative books on the Alexander Technique

Bacci, Ingrid, *The Art of Effortless Living,* Perigee Books 2002.

Brennan, Richard, *The Alexander Technique Manual,* Little Brown 1996.

Brennan, Richard, *Mind and Body Stress Relief with the Alexander Technique,* Thorsons 1996.

Brennan, Richard, *The Alexander Technique – New Perspectives,* Chrysalis Books 2001.

Brennan, Richard, *Improve Your Posture with the Alexander Technique,* Duncan Baird Publishers 2010.

Chance, Jeremy, *The Alexander Technique,* Thorsons 1998.

Gelb, Michael, *Body Learning,* Aurum Press 1981.

Nicholls, Carolyn, *Body, Breath and Being,* D & B Publishing 2008.

Park, Glen, *The Art of Changing,* Ashgrove Press 1989.

Stevens, Chris, *The Alexander Technique,* Optima 1987.

Westfeldt, Lulie, *F. Matthias Alexander –The Man and His Work,* Centerline Press 1964.

More in-depth or specialized books on the Alexander Technique

Balk, Malcolm, and Andrew Shields, *Master the Art of Running,* Collins & Brown 2009.

Barlow, Marjorie, *An Examined Life,* Mornum Time Press 2002.

Barlow, Wilfred, *The Alexander Principle,* Gollancz 1973.

Carrington, Walter, *Thinking Aloud,* Mornum Time Press 1994.

Conable, Barbara, *How to Learn the Alexander Technique,* Andover Press 1991.

Heirich, Jane, *Voice and the Alexander Technique,* Mornum Time Press 2004.

Macdonald, Patrick, The *Alexander Technique as I See It,* Sussex Academic Press 1989.

Maisel, Edward, *The Resurrection of the Body,* Shambala 1969.

Pierce Jones, Frank, *The Freedom to Change – The Development and Science of the Alexander Technique,* Mouritz 1997.

Shaw, Stephen, *Master the Art of Swimming,* Collins & Brown 2009.

Vineyard, Missy, *How You Stand, How You Move, How You Live,* Morlowe and Company 2007.

Books by F.M. Alexander himself

Alexander, F.M., *The Use of the Self,* Gollancz 1985.

Alexander, F.M., *The Universal Constant in Living,* Centerline Press 1986.

Alexander, F.M., *Constructive Conscious Control of the Individual,* Gollancz 1987.

Alexander, F.M., *Man's Supreme Inheritance,* Centerline Press 1988.

Other books by Richard Brennan

The Alexander Technique – Natural Poise for Health, Vega Books 2003

The Alexander Technique Manual, Little, Brown 1996

Mind & Body Stress Relief with the Alexander Technique, Thorsons 1998

Stress – The Alternative Solution, Foulsham 2000

References

Alexander, F.M., *The Use of the Self*, Gollancz 1985.

Alexander, F.M., *The Universal Constant in Living*, Centerline Press 1986.

Alexander, F.M., *Constructive Conscious Control of the Individual*, Gollancz 1987.

Alexander, F.M., *Man's Supreme Inheritance*, Centerline Press 1988.

Barlow, Wilfred, *The Alexander Principle*, Gollancz 1973.

Bronowski, Jacob, *The Ascent of Man*, BBC Books 1973.

Conable, Barbara, *How to Learn the Alexander Technique*, Andover Press 1991.

Garlick, David, *The Lost Sixth Sense – A Medical Scientist Looks at the Alexander Technique*, Centatime 1990.

Huxley, Aldous, *Means and Ends*, Chatto and Windus 1937.

Anaïs Nin, *The Diary of Anaïs Nin*, vol. 4, Harcourt 1971.

Pierce Jones, Frank, *The Freedom to Change – The Development and Science of the Alexander Technique*, Mouritz 1997.

Shaw, George Bernard, *London Music in 1888–1889 as Heard by Corno di Bassetto (later known as Bernard Shaw) with some Further Autobiographical Particulars*, Dodd, Mead 1937.

Spencer, Herbert, *The Principles of Ethics*, Liberty Classics 1978.

Tinbergen, Nikolaas, transcript of Nobel Prize Winner's acceptance speech, *Science*, 185: 20–27, 1974.

Tolle, Eckhart, *A New Earth – Awakening to Your Life's Purpose*, Penguin 2006.

Acknowledgements

There are many people I would like to thank for making the production of this book possible. First of all, Susan Mears and Michael Mann of Element books, and friend and freelance editor Sarah Widdicombe, who were so encouraging and helpful producing the first edition of the workbook. Secondly, Katie Cowan, Caroline King, Jane Birch, Martin Hendry, Caroline Molloy, Gemma Wilson, Mike Parsons, Melissa Spencer, Tim Brennan and Mckinley Blake for all their help in producing this edition. Thirdly, Dr Miriam Wohl, Dr Andrew Glaister and Jane Heirich, who gave me helpful ideas on how to improve on the original book. Next, all my Alexander teachers over the years who have taught me everything I know: Danny Reilly, Jean McGowan, Trish Hemmingway, Danny McGowan, Jeanne Haahr, Jorgen Haahr, Paul Collins, Chris Stevens, Alan Mars, Refia Sacks, David Gorman, Tommy Thompson, Michaela Wohlgemuth and Giora Pinkas. Also, all my pupils and students who I learn so much from. I would also like to thank my wife and greatest friend, Caroline, who supported me by looking after the house and family, whose talents included creating and taking care of my website! Lastly, I would also like to thank all those readers who over the years have sent me letters and e-mails of thanks for the original workbook.

Photography credits:

All photography by Caroline Molloy, except p16 and 38: Getty Images; p21: F. M. Alexander

Index